Uncovering the Treasure

CLASSICAL TAI CHI'S PATH TO INTERNAL ENERGY & HEALTH

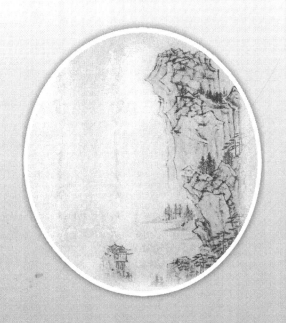

Stephen Hwa, Ph. D.

ISBN: 1449917895
ISBN-13: 9781449917890

Library of Congress Control Number: 2009912895

Acknowledgements

I would like to thank my wife, Eva. It was her urging and encouragement that convinced me to work on my Tai Chi DVDs and now this book. Her help in preparing this manuscript was invaluable. I want to thank Sifu Jim Roach and Tom Kostusiak of our Buffalo school for participating in many of the demonstration photos included in this book. I am grateful to Master Sonia Young for stepping in and teaching me, at times, during the absence of Grandmaster Young Wabu.

Thanks to my student, Joe Milne, for compiling the 108 Form Names. I want to thank Sensei Faust of Faust's USA Karate, where I teach my Tai Chi classes, for her constant support. I want to thank all my students in class and distance, through whom many of the discussions in this book became crystallized.

This book is dedicated to

Grandmaster Young Wabu
and his teacher,
Grandmaster Wu Chien Chuan

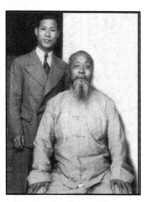

Young Wabu, at left, and Grandmaster Wu Chien Chuan, taken at Young's residence in Kowloon.

CONTENTS

Chapter VIII (cont.)

Chapter IX

Chapter X

Chapter XI

Appendix

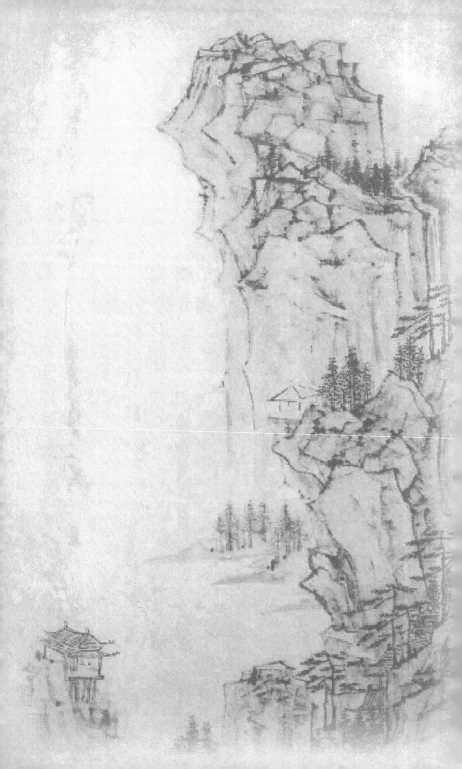

INTRODUCTION

There are so many books, classes, and styles of tai chi today. In many of them, there is talk of internal energy yet the definition is vague and the route to achieving it left unexplained.

Join me in uncovering the crucial missing pieces to truly understanding Tai Chi, i.e., the internal energy that powers Tai Chi movements and the learning program to develop such energy. How various components in the Tai Chi teaching program, such as Large Frame and Compact Frame Form, Square and Round Form, silk reeling exercises, etc. fit into the learning program are discussed in detail. It will show that Tai Chi's ability to mobilize the body's energy and deliver it efficiently is one of the prime reasons that distinguish it as a martial art. It is the cultivation of this internal energy that produces the most significant health benefits of Tai Chi.

The other topic discussed in great detail in this book is the body structure or alignment in Tai Chi Form and its applications. Proper body structure or alignment is essential to the mobilization and delivery of energy and qi flow. It is also essential to maintaining healthy joints in the body for the long haul. Therefore, some of these discussions delve deep into the nitty-gritty of the movements not usually seen in other Tai Chi books which usually emphasize the ethereal aspects of Tai Chi.

I sense there is an unspoken belief among modern Tai Chi practitioner that as long as one has the right mental state, almost any movement is a Tai Chi movement. As a result, infinite varieties of Tai Chi Forms sprout everywhere. Those early Masters who developed Classical Tai Chi Form must have had in depth knowledge about body mechanics and its effect on joint health and energy transmission and generation in the body. They meticulously incorporated their knowledge into every move in the Tai Chi Form. After all, a bad posture will stop internal energy generation and qi flow. No mental state or wishful thinking can overcome that. That is the reason why I pay so much attention to the details of the movements in the discussion.

Material in this book is based on the teaching from my teacher Young Wabu, who was a student of the legendary master Wu Chien Chuan. From the beginning, I was attracted to Young's teaching not only for its impact on my body's well being but also for the logical, rational and scientific approach. Thirty years of studying this art is truly a road of discovery. I am constantly surprised by discoveries of its benefits, its power, and its exquisite structure created by Masters of the past.

At first glance, it appears to be very complex, but gradually it becomes simpler because every element in it, no matter how minor it is, follows certain rules and these rules form a logical structure with calculated, scientific reasoning behind it. Every element is optimized toward two objectives; martial art applications and health benefits. As a result, every element is tightly coupled with other elements even though they may appear to be unrelated. The entire structure is rooted in Chinese philosophy. It is truly a world heritage treasure.

My attempt to present this treasure to the public first started with the Classical Tai Chi DVD series (www.classicaltaichi.com) and now with this book. Each medium has its advantages and disadvantages. Hopefully, they will complement each other to provide a worthy representation of this treasure.

In this book, I present both the overriding principles and certain individual movements. It is from these individual movements that one can see the connections between different elements and how they fit into the overall schemes. Every one of these movements has sufficient descriptions so that the reader might be able to duplicate the move to test its implications themselves.

I am very curious on when, by whom, and how this exquisite art was developed. It would be such an interesting and illuminating story. Unfortunately this is not to be. Despite many people's efforts at searching, the development of this art remains a mystery. To me, the most reliable information is what my teacher told me, 'that Wu told him that Wu did not change what they learned from the Yang and insisted that they cannot be changed.' I could see why Wu said that it cannot be changed. With all the interlocking relationships between various elements, any change would result into some collapse of the logical structure. To my thinking, if Wu said that it has not been changed after they learned from Yang, I have to trust that statement. Who will not point out their contribution to the art? It is known that Yang Luchan, the founder of Yang style, learned from the 14th generation of the Chen Family, Chen Chang-hsing. But, research indicates that Chen Chang-hsing learned Tai Chi from an outsider, Jiang Fa, which make sense since the Chen family's own famous Canon Chuan (Canon Fist) is based on principles opposite to what was taught by Wu's. Beyond this point the history becomes vague. In the brief record available to us, none gets into the specifics so that one could get a sense of how it was perfected.

We can only celebrate what is transmitted from Wu Chien Chuan and the good fortune that the turmoil of war brought Wu to Hong Kong. Wu appreciated Young's natural ability and his dedication by discarding completely the external martial arts for which Young was known. Wu was willing to stay at Young's home to teach him. They worked night and day with very little distraction. This is reflected in the rigorous and in-depth material that is passed on. If Young had sought Wu as a teacher at Wu's home base in Shanghai, he would not have such dedicated attention since Wu was a much sought after teacher with many students there. For this, we should be thankful for what fate brought about.

CHAPTER 1:

INTERNAL DISCIPLINE OF TAI CHI

The eventual goals of learning tai chi are often described as:

- Using internal movement to direct external motion 以内形的運轉來支配外形的動作 is the foundation of Tai Chi's Internal Discipline (neigong).
- During Form playing, the external appears to be soft and relaxed, while internally neijing (internal energy) is created and circulates throughout the body. 外柔内剛，勁蘊於内 This is the origin of Tai Chi's health benefits and power for martial art applications
- Incorporate Internal Discipline (neigong) into every Tai Chi Form movement. 太極内功蘊藏在拳架中.

Thus, Form practice is the way to develop internal energy for martial art applications and tune the body to achieve the ideal of "live forever in the spring season of your life".

Internal Discipline is sometimes called "Torso Method". Jou, Tsung Hwa in his celebrated treatise, "THE TAO

OF TAI-CHI CHUAN: Way to Rejuvenation", Tai Chi Foundation, 1991, page A31, stated that "The Second Stage. The hallmark of the second stage is the use of torso method. Torso method is characterized by use of the body, specifically the waist and spine, to initiate and empower the movements of the arms and legs. .... Only those who reach this stage can truly be said to be practicing Tai Chi, yet these are few indeed."

The most important instruction on Internal Discipline passed down from Wu Chien Chuan to my teacher Young Wabu is "Every movement in Tai Chi Form has to have two complementary parts of the body, a moving part (called the yang part) and a stationary part (called yin part). When the yin-yang junction is located in the torso of the body, it is an internal move. When it is outside of the torso, it is an external move." This seemingly simple and unremarkable statement has tremendous implications on many aspects of Tai Chi. At this point, I want to just mention two important contributions from this statement: One is that this statement is the key to a methodology that enables Tai Chi practitioners to mobilize the powerful core of the body for Tai Chi movements, to generate internal energy and internal energy circulation in the body. The other is the health benefits. From a health benefits viewpoint, movements using internal discipline penetrate to the deep recesses of the torso, stimulating and invigorating the organs and the circulatory systems in the torso. The body is further benefited from the circulating internal energy and 'qi' during Form playing. It is the primary reason why Tai Chi will enhance the robustness of the body's internal systems.

Examples of Moves Using Internal Discipline

Turning

Try to stand with two feet parallel to each other, about shoulder-width apart. Then, turn the body without moving the feet. Most people who have not been trained in Classical Tai Chi, will turn at the hip carrying the torso with it, while the legs will have a twisting motion following the hip. see Picture 1-1. This is a weak external move without much power and the body structure has poor balance and stability. In Classical Tai Chi, the turning move is carried out at the waist using the power of the abdomen and back, while the pelvis and the legs essentially are not moving , providing a stable framework and grounding. see Picture 1-2 & 1-3. When this move is done correctly, a strong internal energy flow in the waist region can be felt. One can classify this move as a half body move-upper half vs. lower half of the body. The upper body is yang (moving) while the lower body is yin (not moving). The yin-yang junction is at the waist.

For the beginner, the difficulty lies in the mental discipline in which all attention has to be concentrated on the core region. Any attention on the shoulder and the turning move will be partially initiated from the shoulder. One can see whether or not the shoulder is involved by doing the move in front of a mirror. When it is done correctly, there should be no sensation feedback from shoulder and arm. The yang part of the body, i.e. upper chest, shoulder and arm, is relaxed, just following the move of the waist. Within the yin part of the body, on the other hand, there are some complex, small and powerful moves. The portion of the core just above the pelvis, together with the buttocks, exerts a counter twist to the pelvis to keep the pelvis stable. In other words, the upper abdominal muscle turns in one direction carrying the yang part of the body while the lower abdominal muscle turns slightly to the other direction to stabilize the pelvis. (see Picture I-4 & I-5).

Folding

The folding move involves one entire side of the body; arm, torso, and leg, moving as a unit. In the example shown in Picture I-6 & I-7, the left side of the body is folding or unfolding by keeping the right side of the body stationary. The stationary part provides support, some of the power for the move, and grounding. The left side of the body is yang, the right side of the body is yin. The yin-yang junction is at the spine. One can visualize that the spine is a hinge, so each side of the body, like a door, can fold or unfold using that hinge. This is also a half -body move, right side vs. left.

This move in Tai Chi classics is described as "upper and lower body following each other" 上下相隨

Another classical description is, " hand follows the foot, elbow follows the knee, and shoulder follows the hip". This is an important example of how to make a move but still keep each side of the body's alignment intact. This move can be achieved only when the turning power comes from the waist and the entire back's muscles. If one uses the upper body power for this move, the lower body will not likely be able to follow upper body's move. The left foot will likely be lagging behind the move to form a twisted structure on the left side of the body, greatly reducing the power of the move.

Lift Leg
Lift the left leg by using abdominal and back muscles to lift the left side of the pelvis which in turn lifts the leg. In this case, the left leg is completely relaxed since the lifting is done by internal power not the leg muscle. The moving part is the left leg and

its associated abdominal and back muscles while the other parts of the body remain stationary to provide support and grounding. The yin-yang junction may be visualized in the left abdominal and back region. One could classify this as a lower left, quarter -body move.

All lower body movements are from the core. This is just one example of it. Practicing with an imaginary mental picture that the legs do not end at the hip joints, but rather, there is a leg extension into the core of the body has helped some students learn how to initiate lower body movements from the core.

Hand Push Forward

Instead of stretching the right hand out from the shoulder and elbow, which is an external move, one can mobilize the abdominal and back muscles to push out the right, upper chest, shoulder and arm while the rest of the stationary body supports the move, connects the move to ground, and provides a substantial portion of the power for the move. In this case, the yang part of the body, right chest, shoulder and arm, is relaxed without strain, since all the work is done internally (see Picture I-8). The yin-yang junction can be considered in the region around right side of the torso. One can see the change in the crease of the shirt showing the abdominal muscle movement in Picture 1-9 & 1-10. This is classified as an upper right, quarter-body move.

This is a typical 'fajin' move, a very short stroke, forward move, with a sudden burst of power. This move is by far more difficult to master than the previous three moves. One of the difficulties is that most people have deeply ingrained habits of stretching the arm out from shoulder and elbow. It is necessary to first train them to keep the arm and shoulder quiet without moving before teaching them the internal move. To stop students from making habitually bad movements is often more difficult than teaching them to make the right movements.

Again, the yang part of the body is relaxed without strain while the yin part of the body has complex, small and powerful movements. For example, the forward thrust developed by the core generates an opposite force or reaction force. One can easily see how this reaction force is transmitted through the leg to be absorbed by the ground in a small but visible wave traveling from the buttock downward along that leg on the same side of the body as the forward-pushing arm.

When one tries to learn the four moves discussed above, it is important to keep the simple, idealized picture as described in the first paragraph of each move in mind and not to be concerned with other details of the move. This is the general methodology of learning: always keep a simple mental picture of how the yin-yang segments in the torso move relative to each other even though such an idealized picture is only an approximation. Over time, with long practice, this picture will guide the move toward the intended goal.

When one carries out an internal move, the power of the move is primarily from the abdomen and the back muscles, while the muscle of the moving (yang) part is relaxed. When done correctly, one will feel the sensation of stretching and intense energy generation across the yin-yang boundary in the torso. All my students have reported that this is a very enjoyable sensation. In fact, it is one of the driving forces of keeping them trying even though it is demanding to learn, both mentally and physically.

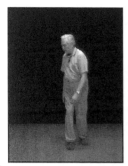
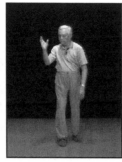
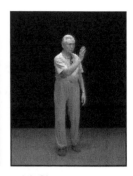

(Picture I-1, Picture I-2, Picture I-3)

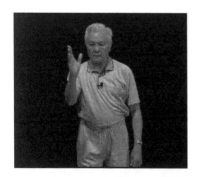
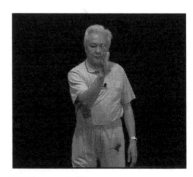

(Picture I-4 and Picture I-5)

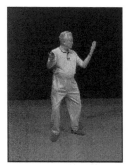 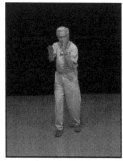 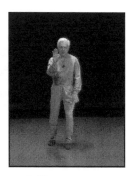

(Picture 1-6, Picture 1-7, Picture 1-8)

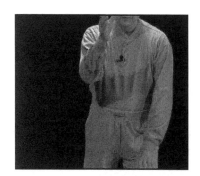 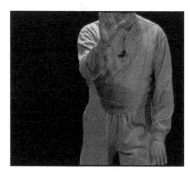

(Picture 1-9 and Picture 1-10)

CHAPTER 11:

BENEFITS OF PRACTICING TAI CHI
WITH INTERNAL DISCIPLINE

Every aspect of Tai Chi Form practice has to satisfy two requirements simultaneously; 1) It has to be useful for martial art applications. 2) It has to be useful for health benefits. Classical Tai Chi Form accomplishes these goals superbly. For example, playing the Tai Chi with Internal Discipline fully utilizes the powerful core of the body, the abdomen and the back. It is also a uniquely effective means of invigorating the internal organs and the circulatory and nervous systems.

Martial Art Applications
The heart of Internal Discipline is mobilizing the energy resources of the body in the most optimal way. Since the core muscles, when coordinated properly, are the most versatile and powerful muscle group in the body, they should play a central role in energy generation. When one examines the best power move in any sport, a majority of them use the principle of Internal

Discipline. When this power mobilization process is incorporated into Form movements which are designed based on martial art considerations, it becomes a martial art move with a stored energy surge ready to be released. "Store energy like a fully drawn bow, release energy like releasing an arrow 蓄勁如張弓　發勁如放箭

During Form playing, the internal energy circulates continuously in the torso of the body without release. But, during martial applications, the internal energy will surge out to the opponent through the limbs, hands or legs, or through body contact such as the shoulder. It is sometime called fajin or fajing. To utilize this energy effectively in martial applications, one has to master the art of applications - strategy, tactics, and finesse. Some of these are unique to tai chi, such as: sticking to the opponent, following rather than resisting the opponent's force, trapping (such as when an opponent is coming low at you make him go lower), using four ounces of force to deflect a thousand pounds of incoming force, soft conquering hard, and etc. To sum up, find the opponent's weak point then counterattack with the delivery of the internal energy or fajin.

The art of applications; strategy, tactics, and finesse is steeped in Chinese philosophy. It is extensively discussed in tai chi classics as well as in all recent tai chi publications. To actually develop this art requires long practice of push hands and sparring exercises where "give and take" with an opponent is essential. On the other hand, practicing Tai Chi Form with Internal Discipline develops internal energy or power, trains the body to move correctly and with the right body structure, building a solid foundation in the body before tackling the "two bodies" challenge. Since most Tai Chi Form practiced today lacks the element of Internal Discipline and proper body structure, it has lost its worth and gradually been de-emphasized. On one hand, there are the schools that emphasize sparring, push hands and weapons practice, neglecting the Form, without knowing that the Form builds the internal energy and power for martial arts application. On the other hand, are schools that say one must do the Forms but also alongside, one must separately practice qi gong exercises. Ironically, practicing the Forms with Internal Discipline inherently is an excellent qi gong exercise! Learning Classical Tai Chi Form with internal discipline requires concentration and patience. And yet, there are rich rewards in every step of the way whether the student is a beginner or advanced practitioner.

Health Benefits

An early Tai Chi master once wrote that the ultimate purpose of learning Tai Chi was 'to live forever in the spring season of your life". Tai Chi is not just for longevity, but also for robustness through old age.

The health benefits of Classical Tai Chi may be viewed from several different angles and at different levels, all of which tie in strongly with the practice of Internal Discipline.

When examining the movements of very young children, we see that the movements of their arms and legs often originate from the torso. Their movements are relaxed and without tension. As we grow older, our movements tend to concentrate on our arms, legs and shoulders and less on our torso. Also, tension and stiffness start to creep into our movements. Gradually, we lose touch with our torso. Eventually, stagnation of the torso sets in. We often see the elderly walking with a shuffle—the walking movement no longer extends into the torso. With all the major organs and complex circulatory system residing in the torso, it's easy to understand the adverse effect of inaction and stagnation of the torso on the health of the body. One may assert that the onset of internal rigor mortis actually precedes death!

Classical Tai Chi may be considered as a means to return to childhood. Movements using Internal Discipline penetrate to the deep recesses of the torso, stimulating and invigorating the organs and the circulatory systems in the torso. For example, the fluids in the lymphatic system needs body movement to pump its circulation. Enhancement of the function of the intestine and kidney are immediate; while impact on other organs is more long term. Integrating Internal Discipline in everyday life not just during Form practice would be most effective in achieving a healthy life style.

Modern exercise routines, including martial arts, are long on external movements and short on internal movements. In other words, exercise the parts of the body which are already over-used for an active person while neglect the portion of the body which needs exercise. Worse yet, these routines often subject the shoulder, knee, the back and other joints with ill-conceived repetitive, unnatural movements. No wonder many active people eventually develop joint problems. Classical Tai Chi, through the experience of multi-generations of practitioners who practice from a young age until the end of life, fully grasp the importance of proper postures and movements to protect and strengthen the joints for long term, repetitive practice. For example, part of the reason for the "folding move" discussed before, is to keep the lag and that side of the body aligned during movement to minimize any shear force or twist in the knee joint and hip joint. "Knee should not project beyond the toe" is a very important and strictly enforced rule, again to prevent over extension injury to the knee. "Turn the hip slightly forward to avoid the buttocks stick out from behind" and "stretching the head up" are both intended to maintain the health of the spine. Many movements are beneficial to the health of spine. As a result, beginning practitioners often cite reduced or eliminated lower back pain and weakness as the first benefits of practicing Classical Tai Chi. To keep the integrity and mobility of the body structure during movements is an important topic in almost every thread of discussion in this book.

The movement of pushing the arm forward, as discussed before, the elbow points downward and stays in front of the body. In this way, the arm is solidly braced so it can deliver the powerful internal energy to an opponent without buckling during martial arts application. The position of the elbow also protects the mid-portion of the body. From a health viewpoint, this movement fully stretches and relaxes the upper back, tuning and strengthening it. Those who have pain in their upper back often find that playing the Tai Chi form alleviates their problem. Throughout the Tai Chi form movements, the synergy between martial art and health is spontaneous and natural without coercion.

Practicing tai chi moves with Internal Discipline is physically and mentally very taxing for a beginner irrespective whether or not this person has a strong body. When their training advances, their internal energy gets stronger, and yet they will feel more effortless in doing the movements. In other words, one has built up internal robustness. As long as one continues Tai Chi practice every day, one will retain or even improve robustness with age. This is what "live forever in the spring season of your life" means.

Applications of Internal Discipline Other Than Martial Arts

Classical Tai Chi Form takes a balanced approach toward tight coupling with martial arts application and broad applications outside of martial arts. My Tai Chi friend in Shanghai, Master Yuanyi, showed me the Tai Chi Form from his lineage which is a total integration with push hands. It anticipates moves from an opponent during push hands and the Form movements were designed accordingly. It is very sophisticated with great subtlety. It is also very specialized in its applications. Comparatively, Classical Tai chi Form is much more centered on the practitioner not on the potential opponent. It develops internal energy or power, trains the body to move correctly and with the right body structure, building a solid foundation in one's own body before tackling the challenge from an opponent. The result is that it can be adopted for broad applications outside of martial arts. My students are encouraged to apply what they learn to everyday life. This will accelerate their learning of Internal Discipline and also enjoy the benefits from it.

It is also beneficial to everyday life when one wants to use one's power to do any chore. Integrating Internal

Discipline into everyday life is the best way to master the art rapidly.

My students often report to me about how they apply what they learned.

Bill is a kitchen cabinet installer. He often mentioned that he applies what he learned in Tai Chi to his work which has made his job physically much easier on him.

Marie worked in a university. Her workplace had spring loaded doors which were very difficult to open. When she tried to use the turning internal move to open the door, the door opened so easily that it almost hit her head.

Mike is a bass player. He finds that by introducing more core movement into the bowing action in place of the arm movement, he can get a better sound out of his instrument.

Greg is a ski instructor. He is often surprised at how the principles in Classical Tai Chi agree with the principles of skiing. Many of my students apply "Tai Chi Walk" principles when they are walking on icy road surfaces. Certainly, Internal Discipline will be a very useful training for sports applications. If one watches the actions of most professional athletes, one finds that athletes know how to use the core well while most amateurs do not. In other words, after years of practice of several moves relevant to their sports, a few people learn how to utilize their core very well and they rise to the top of their sport. But, most of them reach this stage through their talent rather than through a well designed internal power training program. One often hears the coach admonish the player, "use your body, not just your arm". The coach can see the problem in the player but does not have an approach to teach them how to use the body, not just the arm. I believe one can tailor Internal Discipline training for specific sports so that using core power optimally can be trained systematically.

I was a tennis player since a very young age. My game started going downhill when I was approaching forty years of age. That was when I started to learn Tai Chi. As I was beginning to master the Internal Discipline in my Tai Chi Form practice in my fifties, my tennis game started to improve rapidly. It eventually reached a level way beyond my younger years. Take some specific moves as examples: I did not learn the proper technique to volley at the net when I was young. Later, I found my upper quarter-body push move is exactly the correct move for a volley, described by tennis pros as a "punch" move. The body turning move in "Grasp Peacock's Tail" greatly improved my two-handed backhand. Overall, my moves were much more natural, powerful and I had a faster response on the court, as if I had rebuilt myself from ground up into an entirely different person with physical and mental abilities beyond my youthful years.

CHAPTER III:

EVOLVEMENT OF MIND – BODY RELATIONSHIP DURING THE LEARNING PROCESS

Mental state of a beginner

We think about dexterity of hands or feet but think of the torso as a dull part of the body, not knowing that the torso can be developed to have just as much dexterity. As a result, almost everyone who starts on Classical Tai Chi is awkward in their torso. Precise command and control of the neuromuscular system in the torso area are nonexistent. Yet, it is crucial in the development of Internal Discipline. During early Form training, students have to look intensely inward trying to establish communication with the torso, not just for command and control but also to develop sensitivity to the sensation of the body's feedback. Knowing the correct sensation of a movement is one of the best tools to achieve self-improvement. It is a very rewarding exercise when one can sense the gradual discoveries of his own body which has been hidden all these years. This also has important health implications. In China, a healthy and well-tuned nervous system is considered to be paramount to a healthy body. If the nervous system at certain parts of the body is dull and irresponsive, health problems are usually not far away.

Overcoming mental blockage is the major task in the tai chi learning process. Sometimes it is not useful to just tell students "you have to be relaxed in these places". Students just do not have the neuromuscular control to do it. The teaching program in the sections below on tai chi Form emphasizes a step by step approach to gradually ease into the more difficult situations.

Yi-Martial Art Intention

Most people are learning Tai Chi probably for reasons other than for serious martial art applications. So the question is how much should we emphasize the martial art aspects of Tai Chi? Certainly Tai Chi Form movements make more sense and are easier to remember if they are corroborated by the martial arts origin of the movements - why there are these sequences of movements, and what the positioning of body and timing of the movements mean. Besides this aspect, there is a more subtle but powerful reason why the martial arts aspect of Tai Chi is important.

Tai Chi Form should be practiced with "Yi" (martial art intention). "Yi" is not something complex and elaborate. It is single minded and somewhat intuitive with the desire to deliver the internal power externally through hands, arm and foot, whatever the movement is. If the hand is moving forward, then the Yi goes to the palm and fingers; if the hand is moving laterally in a blocking movement, then the Yi goes to the leading edge on the side of the hand, etc. Once the practitioner masters the "Yi", it is no long a conscious effort any more. It becomes subconscious and comes naturally whenever the practitioner makes a move. At this stage, when you play the Form, you have both the internal energy and qi (nerve signal, a simple-minded definition) circulating in the torso of your body. With the "Yi" as a catalyst, the qi is able to flow to your hands and fingers. A small portion of the internal energy also follows qi flow to the fingers. The majority of the internal energy continues to circulate in your torso until you need it for an application. Then, this portion of the internal energy will follow the qi to the arms, hands, and fingers for delivery.

External martial arts such as Karate also practice a solo form called Kata. Kata allows the practitioner to study movements at full power and speed and allows the student to move with the enemy in mind. So, both Tai Chi form and Kata is practiced with "Yi". But, Kata is practiced with a tensed-up arm moving with power and speed while Tai Chi is practiced with a relaxed arm and moving at a slow speed. The "Yi" in Tai Chi is therefore purely mental.

For some students, "Yi" is fairly easy to develop. It is almost natural to them. For some students, it is quite difficult to be consistent – other intentions creep in subconsciously from time to time. Students who have studied dancing or are interested in dancing sometimes have such problems. Normally, the fingers become very warm after playing the Form even in cold weather. One of my students who had already achieved good internal movements complained about cold fingers. Upon close examination, she frequently had small, unnecessary flourishes in her hands and fingers. After reducing that flourish, her problem of cold fingers improved. Extraneous motions, or nerve signals, along the path of qi, such as shoulder, elbow, and arms, have the same effect of disrupting the flow of qi between the body and the fingers. People who use their hands intensively, such as dancers, typists, and piano players could have such problems. It is important for them to keep localized nerve activity dormant and let the qi from the body take over. This is a good reason to learn the Square Form from which the practitioner will get used to movements with steady arms and hands without localized impulses.

The focus here is on the arms and hands, not on the legs and feet. The reason is that during form playing, the lower limbs have definite functions to perform and their energy and qi are already integrated with that of the torso. During Form playing, the upper limb's function is entirely abstract and mental and is easily distracted.

The above discussion of Yi was initially published on the Classical Tai Chi Student's Forum. One of the students, Barbara R., posted an interesting response which is copied below:

"I found Master Hwa's discussion of yi and cold hands and dancers' problems in taking up tai chi interesting because of my own experience. When I used to do ballet, the palm side of my hands and fingers would get very warm and flushed and so would my teacher's. As she was older and had high blood pressure and none of the other students seemed bothered by "hot hands," it really kind of worried me a little. When I started doing tai chi and found out warmth and flush and tingling in the hands could all be signs of chi flowing correctly, I was relieved in retrospect, but disappointed, because I didn't have any of those experiences playing the form. I thought maybe it was because of so much keyboarding in the years between—enough to cause some carpal tunnel syndrome problems. Then, in the last few months, I began to have some color and tingling while practicing and hoped it was some healing effect taking place. Master Hwa's piece offers another explanation.

When I first started doing tai chi, I had no idea what most of the motions were for. Since then, I've learned a good bit more about applications and now often play the form to an audience of imaginary opponents "walking the circle" around me like ba gua players. (That is the way to practice- Master Hwa) This is actually much nearer the way I used to practice ballet--with the intent of expressing to an audience, real or imaginary, whatever character or emotion the dance I was doing was supposed to represent.

The "yi" in ballet--mind intent if not martial intent--seems to come in with the desire to project ("To Project" is the key- Master Hwa); so maybe it is learning about the martial applications that's making my tai chi playing better for me."

Certain segments of the population want to learn tai chi but are turned off by its association with martial arts. Barbara again has some interesting observation:

"I think that women in the west even today often have a problem in perceiving fighting skills as being "artistic" enough to be appropriate for them because of the way they are often depicted in our culture and because of a tendency in the culture itself to label "art" as being more of a woman's thing than a man's and "defending" as being a masculine prerogative. ... I can't think of any fighting skill in western culture that has anything like the same cachet of art and beauty about it.....Maybe one of the reasons I was drawn to Wu style was Wu Ying Hua and Wu Yan Hsia, Master Young's daughter (Sonia Young, all three are accomplished women Tai Chi Master-Master Hwa)...........

I think the biggest help is to find something in the martial essence of tai chi that you can relate to and use it as a bridge to the rest. For me, maybe one of the best is something I read recently about peng (I think you mean teng jin, which means listening to opponent's jin(power) -Master Hwa).

I certainly ought to be able to relate to that, after spending so much time walking herding breed dogs off leash and having to "listen" to their muscle tension and for anything about to come our way so as to be able to "ward off" their attacks on cars and cats before they start. That may sound bizarre, but just as you mentioned applying the principles of tai chi to everyday life, I think you have to find your point of entry to a martial arts mindset, if it seems alien to you, wherever you can."

Progressing From Beginner to Advanced Practitioner

The first stage is to reclaim one's body as one's own so that the torso no longer ignores the commands to make a move. One begins to be able to make differentiation between energized parts of the body and relaxed parts of the body: yang (moving) and yin (non-moving). The indications are that in order to achieve true relaxation, one may have to achieve some energizing first, so that attention could concentrate on the energized not on the relaxed. When one has no intent on certain parts of the body and no feedback sensation from these parts, these parts will achieve true relaxation. My student Ernie said that trying to relax the shoulder did not work for him, because the act of "trying to relax" placed too much attention on the shoulder which kept the shoulder in play. But, this is a chicken and egg problem. Energizing and energy flow thrive in a relaxed body. Any tenseness impedes the mobilization and flow of energy. Obviously, there is no quick way to achieve energizing and relaxation simultaneously in the body but practice, practice.

One can now perform the choreographic moves of the form. As far as internal moves, internal move controlled lower body and legs, will come first. Upper body internal moves are more difficult. As pointed out earlier, the arm movements are very abstract. The only guide is the martial art intent. Without it, it is just an aimless move while the leg movements have a definite function: supporting the weight and movement of the body. Another important factor is that the core muscles are located right above the pelvic bone which connects to the legs through the hip. It is easier to connect the legs with the core as a unit. The shoulders are located quite a distance away from the core muscles. One could master the internal move using core muscle. But to meld the arm with the core muscle into a single unit capable of delivering the explosive internal energy (fajin) without any loss of power is the holy grail of internal movement.

The eventual goal for Form training is that during form playing, all movements are internal and are fully integrated with the limbs to achieve "using internal movement to direct external motion". Internal energy will circulate in the body continuously without break. At this stage, the advanced practitioner should be able to play the Form without thinking, entirely subconscious. Also, one should be able to integrate internal moves into everyday life, naturally, without effort.

The mind-body relation starting from the intense struggle and engagement of the beginner's stage, progresses to total disengagement. The mind is now free to enjoy the pleasurable sensation of stretching and energy circulation in the body during Form practice as if the mind belongs to an independent observer. This last state of mind is indistinguishable from motion-induced qi gong exercises. This is when Tai Chi and qi gong becomes one.

Tai Chi teaching should not bring emphasis on qi into the teaching program too early which will confuse the already overwhelmed beginner students even more. Some students, halfway into the learning process, because they can already do some internal move and silk reeling exercise, can sense the tingling in their hands, warm fingers, etc. , signs of presence of qi. Enamored by the glamorous and mysterious qi, they start to dabble with the advanced, visualization qi gong exercises, or mind-induced qi gong in contrast to the safe, motion-induced qi gong such as Tai Chi. Without a good qi gong teacher, this may lead into wrong path. Problems could include uncontrollable spasmodic motion or the more serious qi gong psychosis which is now included in the <u>DSM-IV</u> as a culture-bound syndrome. The best approach for the student is to practice Tai Chi Form or silk reeling exercise without any conscious thought or hidden longing about qi gong, just enjoy the sensation of internal energy circulation and let qi come naturally.

Learning Programs

The learning programs discussed below include Tai Chi Forms, silk reeling exercises, off-line exercises, push hands, and sparring exercises. The emphasis will be on Tai Chi Form, in particular, the Compact Form or Small Frame Form in contrast to the Large Frame Form. Tai Chi Classics mentioned the two Forms with the saying, "First learn extended (large) then compact". The differences in characteristics between the two frames are significant, with very different approaches. Within each Frame, there are gradations such as mid-compact and tight-compact. The differences between these variations are less significant. Usually, when a person learns mid-compact he can progress to tight-compact on his own without altering the fundamental approaches.

In the publication, Wu, Kung-tsao (1980, 2006). *Wu Family T'ai Chi Ch'uan* 吳家太極拳, Chien-ch'uan T'ai-chi Ch'uan Association. <u>ISBN 0-9780499-0-X</u>. (sometimes referred to as the Gold Book), Wu Chien

Chuan's Form photos are excellent examples of Large Frame. On the other hand, Wu Kung Yi's photos show a Form more compact. When Wu Chien Chuan taught my teacher, Young Wabu, he started with a Compact Form even more compact than those shown in Wu Kung Yi's photo. The characteristics and its implications of different sizes of the Forms will be examined below.

CHAPTER IV:

LARGE FRAME AND COMPACT FRAME FORMS

The obvious differences in external appearance of the two Frames are the size of the step, the height of the stance, extension of the limbs, and height of the kick. Compact Form uses step size from two and half foot (the actual foot of the person) length (see Picture IV-1), measuring from toe of the front foot to the heel of the back foot, to one and half foot length (see Picture IV-2). The latter is the Tight-Compact Form. All other foot lengths within this range are called Mid-Compact Form. Most of my students feel comfortable at the two foot length, i.e. front heel is about even with back foot's toe. Longer lengths are more suitable for students with longer legs.

Once the step size is selected, two requirements determine the height of the stance, in other words the amount of knee bend:

- Knee never projects over the toe. This is to protect the knee when the weight is on that knee.
- Pelvis faces forward when sitting back. When it is not facing forward that means there is a strong

side and a weak side. An opponent will naturally exploit the weak side. Sitting back and turning is an important move to neutralize and ward off an incoming thrust, and destabilize the opponent. If the body is not facing the opponent squarely, one will not be able to turn the upper body on the weak side sufficiently to be effective. Young said that, in the beginning, Wu constantly wanted him to check this point during sitting back by examining the upper part of both legs to see if they were even with each other (see Picture IV-3). Picture IV-4 shows that when left upper leg is in front of the right, the body is facing right.

The larger the step, the lower one has to sit or lower stance in order to satisfy both these requirements (see Picture IV-6). Wu Chien Chuan's photo show that he did a beautiful job to conform to these rules especially in some very low stance situations, such as the 'low slant flying posture' and the very low 'snake creep down' move. Most other people will have their knee beyond the toe in these situations. The Large Frame has a large step size with low stance, open and extended structure with fully stretched out arms and high kicks with the leg lifting to ninety degrees from vertical. The Compact Form (see Picture IV-5) has a small step size with a high stance, few fully stretched arm moves, and most kicks are carried out at less than forty five degrees aiming at the opponent's shinbone and ankle.

Wu Kung Cho wrote in the Gold Book (page 10) about the Large Frame "Beginners should maintain a low stance so movements unfold in an open and extended fashion. Whether moving forward or backward, make sure that each step alternates unhurriedly between yin and yang. This way, the muscle will gradually become firmer, and the tendon will strengthen. After a long while extending and contracting the joints this way, elasticity begins to develop."   In other words, Large Frame is designed to strengthening external muscles and tendons and to develop a solid lower body foundation. Wu Chien Chuan did not start Young on Large Frame probably because Young was an accomplished external martial artist with a well developed external structure and lower body foundation already.

The difference in appearance described above also signifies the difference in how the movement is accomplished. For example, the large step size and low stance requires the use of leg muscles to push the body forward, backward and upward while the Compact Form primarily use core muscles to pull the body forward and backward. This will be discussed in more detail later. The stretch out and pull back of the arm requires the use of shoulder and arm strength while in the Compact Form, the upper quarter-body movements are entirely internal as discussed previously.

It is difficult to incorporate internal moves and to teach internal discipline to students in the Large Frame

Form, because of its external movements such as the outstretching of arms, large swings of the arm at the shoulders and pushing with the legs. Students will always opt to use the easier external movements. Only when external moves are minimized as in the Compact Form, can internal moves then flourish. Compact Form is single-minded in that every move has to be internal so that when one plays the Form, the internal energy will circulate in the body continuously without break.

The frame size is just one of the two criteria one can use to classify Tai Chi Form. The other criteria is from Square Form to Round Form or from discrete move to continuous move. The following discussion on the Square Form and Round Form are concentrated on Compact Form only.

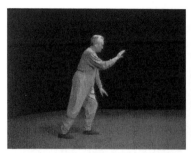 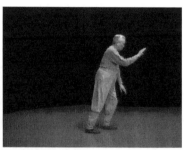

(Picture IV-1 and Picture IV-2)

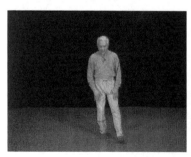 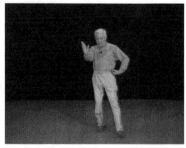

(Picture IV-3 and Picture IV-4)

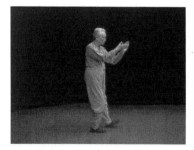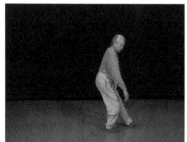

(Picture IV-5 and Picture IV-6)

CHAPTER V:

SQUARE FORM (COMPACT FRAME)

Historically, the Square Form was taught only to the "inner circle" of students who were groomed to be the heirs to the Master's martial arts dynasty. These students were usually the family members of the Masters and a few selected outsiders who served as apprentices to the Masters. I think there are several reasons that the Square Form was not taught to the general student body. Certainly, one was the time availability of the teacher as well as the student, since the learning of the Square Form is time-consuming with many times more moves than the round form to remember. This was true in my own class. Meeting twice a week, students just could not remember all the movements taught in the class. So they could not practice at home. That meant no progress. Now, with the help of video, I find my students relishing the learning of the Square Form. This is like in the old times when the student apprentice was a member of teacher's household with ready access to the teacher. This is also how my teacher Young Wabu learned from his teacher since Wu Chien

Chuan stay at Young's house in Hong Kong. He had his teacher's attention all to himself. Young, who was an exceptional teacher with great patience, firmly believed that all students should start with the Square Form, so I learned the Square Form before the Round Form.

I would like to compare several general characteristics between the Square Form and the Round Form. Not every move in Square Form is internal. It is a preparatory training for the Round Form which is internal in all its movements. Every movement in the Square Form has a clear starting point and ending point with a stop between the moves. The movement between these two points is usually in a straight line and done very crisply and resolutely. Directional changes are usually carried out at these two points. These characteristics are completely opposite to the Round Form, which should have a continuous movement with no apparent starting point or ending point. The hand movements are mostly rounded with few straight-line movements. Therefore, directional changes do not appear at a point rather are incorporated into the movement itself as a smooth curvature. Also the movement in the Round Form, instead of being crisp and resolute should be deliberate and thoughtful. People are often surprised at the directly opposite requirement between the Square Form and the Round Form. Actually, this is not unique. Just think about how one learns the art of calligraphy. One first learns how to write in print form. Then, one learns the cursive form. The differences between these two writing forms are very much analogous to the differences between the two Tai Chi Forms.

The Square Form also avoids the use of upper quarter-body movements and other advanced internal movements. These advanced internal movements will only be taught in the Round Form. As a result, some of the movements in the Square Form are different from the Round Form. In the Round Form, the hand does not make contact with the body. However, there is no such restriction in the Square Form.

In the above discussions, I have emphasized the differences between the Square Form and the Round Form. Actually, there is more sameness than difference.

The Internal Discipline of lower body movements is fully developed in the Square Form. Lower body movements are the foundation of Tai Chi. Poor foot work and poor lower body posture will prevent one from learning Internal Discipline later. It is logical to learn the lower body movements first. In fact, a Square Form lesson by itself is called 'Tai Chi Walk'. This should be the first lesson for student.

Tai Chi Walk

When one demonstrates Tai Chi Form to students, their attention will always be attracted to the upper body movements first and neglect foot works. With this exercise, their attention is forced to be concentrated on the foot works-the foundation of movements. The upper body is kept relaxed with two hands hanging limp on the side of the body. This is the first lesson on how to keep clear a differential between the energized and the relaxed parts of the body working side by side. Even in such simple case, many students have trouble keeping the upper body relaxed in the beginning.

This exercise teaches the proper body posture, feet positions, body weight distribution, and unique walking dynamics. In addition, it is a very effective exercise, tuning every aspect of the lower body including the lower back. Students who have lower back problems often happily report vast improvements once they start on this exercise. The three main characteristics of this exercise are:

1. using core power for leg movements, such as lifting and stretching the leg
2. keeping the body's center of gravity under control, not allowing the body to fall forward as in the common walking motion
3. pulling the body forward or backward not pushing by the leg.

The last move involves primarily the use of the power of the core (described as contracting abdominal muscle inward) together with the pull of the lead foot to move the body. My student, Bill, describe the sensation of this move as if the body is being sucked forward or backward. This is the crucial step for converting the walking motion into an entirely internal movement.

Normally, during walking, one uses the back foot to push when walking forward and the front foot to push when walking backward. The pushing motion by the leg muscle is entirely external and it also engages both feet stuck to the ground until the body completes its move. In other words, it is a double weighted move. In the case of pulling forward instead of pushing forward, the back foot has no responsibility for pushing. It is free to be lifted and moved thereby improving the mobility of the person. The same is true for the backward walk. This is one of the advantages from a martial arts application viewpoint. Certainly during applications, there are situations favoring "push" or situations favoring "pull". For example, when an opponent is coming at you, you want to adhere (stick) to him and sit back to neutralize the incoming force. You certainly do not want to add to his incoming force by pushing your body back with the front foot. Instead, you want to use the back foot and core to control the pull back and at the same time plant the front foot's heel on the ground to absorb some of the incoming force by pulling on the body. "Push" is a natural move and It is further developed and strengthened in the Large Frame Form. On the other hand, "pull" with the core is a learned technique for almost everyone I know and is only developed in the Compact Frame Form.

There are tremendous health benefits associated with the "pull" walking motion. Certainly it improves balance but even more, it stretches the back, strengthens the core region, improving circulation around major internal organs. The benefits of taking a walk are now greatly amplified. For example, I find that after sitting in front of computer for some time, just taking a few steps in this manner, the feeling of stagnation is gone and I feel rejuvenated.

The second characteristic mentioned above "keeping body's center of gravity under control, not allow to fall forward as in the common walking motion" includes a key provision that when one steps out with one foot, the body weight stays back without moving until the front foot is flat on the ground, then one pulls the body forward until all the body weight is on the front foot, while in the common walking motion the body weight shifts with the foot stepping forward so part of the body weight lands on the heels of the front foot. Landing body weight on the heel of the front foot as well as the back foot pushing forward on its toe are the primary reason that people slip and fall on icy or slippery surfaces. Using the walk described eliminates such slips.

In adapting Tai Chi Walk into every day walk, one needs to strip away many of the moves designed to tune the lower body in the Tai Chi Walk lesson and just retain the three characteristics mentioned above as the heart of this exercise. After some practice, one should be able to use it freely for any walking situation. One can now sense the internal energy circulating during walking. It becomes a silk reeling exercise. All my students are encouraged to adopt the Tai Chi Walk for everyday walking.

Once, I was giving a workshop and teaching attendees this walk, one person said "Oh, this is how tribal people walk". I wonder if all humans walked like this when we still lived in an unpaved world. If we didn't, we would all be limping due to stepping into a hole in the grass or slipping on the mud flats.

Square Form as a Template for Round Form

As mentioned before, arm movements are abstract in nature. In the Round Form, with its continuous circular movement, it is difficult to specify or remember movements precisely. Therefore, it is easily corrupted when it is handed over from the teacher to the students. Quite commonly, one sees that students of the same teacher have very different looking Forms. In the Square Form, the continuous circular movement is dissected into many single, straight moves. Each has a definite starting and ending point. The Form learned this way is more precise. The curved movements in the Round Form have to pass through these starting and ending points. Therefore, Square Form provides a template for the Round Form so that it can be handed down through generations with less chance of deviation.

The Concept of Yin (nonmoving) and Yang (moving)

Most untrained people make moves instinctively, not aware how different segments of their body perform different functions in a joint effort to achieve the mission. One of the objectives of Classical Tai Chi is to teach how to identify and then perfect this capability. Square Form is the first step to teach beginners to be familiar with the concept and practice of segmentation. When one part of body moves (yang), the rest of the body is completely still (yin). As discussed before, to achieve internal movements, the yin and yang must be paired to form a junction at the right place in the torso. If there is any movement in the yin, the junction will be altered and result in an entirely different kind of move. That is why when practicing the Square Form the more robotic look, the better. If one does not maintain stillness while other parts of the body move, the object of doing Square Form is compromised.

This is a drill to tune the neuromuscular control of the student. Most beginners cannot keep their neural signals focused on a narrow segment of their body. The diffusion of the signal creates unintended movements. This is called sloppy movements. The correct Square Form movement should look crisp and robotic. To be able to keep part of the body still, by itself, is also important training to eliminate unwanted habitual motions. Sometimes it is more difficult to train students **not** to move than **how** to move.

A good example on the importance of stillness (yin) is the sweeping leg move in which one stands on one leg and sweeps the other leg outward to kick the opponent's feet out from under him. During this move, if the body moves slightly with the sweeping foot, the power of the sweep will diminish. In addition, the knee of the standing foot will feel pain. Since that foot is firmly planted on the ground with the entire body weight on it, any turn of the body above will result in a torque in that knee joint causing pain or injuries (see Picture V-1, V-2, V-3, V-4). In other words, the yin part of the body's alignment has to be instinctively maintained.

The yin-yang pairs practiced in the Square Form are imbedded in the Round Form dynamically transforming from one yin-yang pair to another to give the effect of constant motion and continuity.

The Importance of the Full Stop between Movements

The "stop" or "pause" between moves in the Square Form is a great opportunity for the practitioner to do the following:

- Examine body structure and feet position. Is everything in the right place?
- Enjoy the sensation of stretching, rooting, and energy.

- Prepare for the next move so that it will be carried out with conviction and intent.

All the above functions will have to be carried out in the Round Form on the fly. Here it can be done with all the time needed. Yet, many students become impatient, rushing through the "stop" and resulting in unfocused and weak moves.

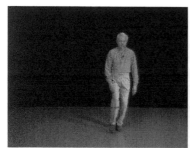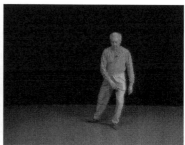

(Picture V-1 and Picture V-2)

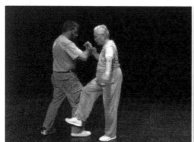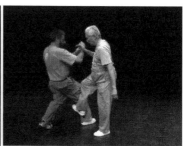

(Picture V-3 and Picture V-4)

CHAPTER VI:

ROUND FORM (COMPACT FRAME)

In class students or distance-learning students (using DVD), those who are well versed in Square Form, adapt to the Round Form quite naturally without the struggle required for starting the Round Form as a beginner. This is because the students now have well tuned neuromuscular control and also a template for the Round Form in mind. The task is now to convert the choreographic (external) moves into internal moves. Compact Round Form is single-minded in that every move has to be internal so eventually when one plays the Form, the internal energy circulates in the body continuously without break. To reach this stage, first, one has to learn how to incorporate Internal Discipline into those important movements which occur repetitively in the Form. Chapter I and Tai Chi Walk already describe several important internal moves in the Form. Several additional ones are described below. In addition to practicing the Form, one should supplement it with silk reeling exercises and offline exercises to learn how to move with internal discipline and enjoy the sensation of internal energy circulation. A way to expedite this learning process to achieve the internal with every move and every transition in the Form will be described later.

Body Forward Lean

A proper forward lean posture requires:

1. All the weight is at the front foot with the front knee bend not projecting beyond the toe
2. Both feet, front and back, are parallel
3. Back foot's heel is firmly on ground
4. Tuck in the behind (or buttock). This requires pressing in the abdominal muscle
5. Head is stretched up in line with the body (see Picture VI-1).

The head, the body and the back leg form a straight line in the lean forward. Under this structure, you will feel a strong stretch from the top of the head down to the Achilles' heel of the back foot. There are numerous times in the 108 Long Form that one moves into this posture from "Brush Knee Push Step", by pressing in the abdominal muscle to pull the body forward (see discussion in Tai Chi Walk). When the "Step" forward move reaches its completion and morphs into the forward lean, the action of the energized abdominal muscle changes to stretching the spine upward and one can sense internal energy flowing upward and downward from the central core region. The body and the back leg forming a straight line, stretched structure provides a straight energy passageway enabling the energy or force flow up and down this passageway without any hindrance.

Our spine is constantly under compression forces due to the action of gravity on the body. I suspect the repetitive stretching of the spine by this move is one of the contributing factors to keeping the body's structure robust even in old age. The up and down energy flow is an important contributor during Form playing to maintaining continuous internal energy circulation.

The forward lean body structure, in the Form, is often associated with the forward push or fajin move. Reaction forces from such fajin moves travel down this energy passageway to be absorbed by the ground without hindrance. If the body structure is perpendicular to the ground with no forward lean, the reaction forces likely would push the body backwards. During sparring, when the opponent pulls, one could forward lean to neutralize the pulling force then counter attack (see Picture VI-2, VI-3, VI-4). The initial power of the counter attack comes from the forward lean structure (Picture VI-2). This "turn body push" move is practiced in the Form such as "Grasp Peacock's Tail" and "Jade Lady Works at the Shuttle". Once the opponent is pushed off balance, the body is readjusted to stick to and pursue the opponent (Picture VI-3 & VI-4).

Many times one sees a person being pulled trying to resist the pulling, struggling to pull back on the opponent which eventually turns into a wrestling match. Many people dislike the forward lean. They feel insecure, as if they will tip over when all weight is on the front leg. With practice this insecure feeling disappears and the body will be relaxed. One will be surprised to find how much forward elongation one can get out of this relaxed body and how much power can be generated at this posture.

The requirements listed above to achieve proper forward lean are common to other moves in the Form and appear to be very simple and yet many students have trouble with them in the beginning. If any one of the requirements is not satisfied, not only will the sensation of stretch and energy flow be absent, but it also will cause the following problems:

- Hesitancy to put all the weight on the front foot, leaving some weight on the back foot results in "double heavy"-Both feet frozen to the ground, unable to move.
- Two feet are not parallel to each other: When forward leaning with the back foot turned outward, the structure not only loses its sensation of stretching but for some people is replaced with a very uncomfortable feeling at the hip joint and the back leg.
- Back foot's heel is not firmly on the ground: when one applies forward fajin on an opponent,

the reaction force will push the heel down first, losing a significant amount of power (this will be further discussed in the section on fajin).

- No tuck in the behind: Eventually may lead to lower back problem.
- Not keeping head, neck, body, and the back leg at a straight line: A major problem for most new students especially those who have studied other styles of Tai Chi before. They will try to straighten the body perpendicular to the ground instead of leaning, or have a knee bent on the back foot, thus the body forms a crescent moon shape instead of a straight line. This weakens the forward fajin power similar to the problem with "heel not on the ground". Also the compression at the lower back is unhealthy to the lower spine. There are reports of a group of tai chi practitioners, practicing such style, all having lower back bone spur problems in their old age. The knee bend of the back leg puts uncomfortable strain on the Achilles tendon and calf muscle, and most likely will result in "heel not on ground".

Students are encouraged to develop a keen sense on the feedback sensation from their body and use such feedback to correct their posture. Any distress signal from any joint indicates something is wrong. I am very surprised to see so many new students are oblivious to such signals and keep on doing the wrong thing. For some, the feedback sensitivity is an acquired ability and needs to be cultivated. If a person is not sensitive to his own body's feedback, he cannot be expected to tien (listen) to another person's jin(power).

The Sit Back Move

In the 108 move Long Form (see attachment), the forward lean move and the sit back move often occur back to back as a yin-yang pair. In push hands exercise, this pair of movements alternate repetitively representing offensive and defensive moves. So, both are extremely important moves in the Form.   During application, when an opponent attacks, stick to opponent, stretch the opponent forward by sitting back, drain some of his forward force, and turn the body to "ward off" to destabilize the opponent.

One starts to practice this move intensely in Tai Chi Walk, and continuous into the rest of the Form practice. Many beginning students consider this move very awkward and therefore do not sit back completely, i.e. not all the body weight rests on the back foot. To do this move correctly, one has to fully tuck the behind in the sitting position so that the backward momentum is absorbed by the tucking motion and then transmitted to the legs. A portion of the momentum can be absorbed by the forward foot with the heel firmly planted on the ground with the tip of the toe drawn up by the stretch in the calf muscle. The forward foot with its heel firmly planted on the ground serves many purposes. It is useful to the balance and stability of the body. It is ready to kick the opponent; to pull the body forward; or to take a step back.

During push hand and Form practice, the sitting back move is often followed by the body moving forward move. To make this transition from "sitting back to moving forward" smooth and effortless, one can take advantage of the stored "sitting back" energy in the forward leg by depressing the toe down with the pelvis drawing the body forward to start the forward motion by pulling with the forward foot. The cycle of back and forward moves can be practiced while waiting in line, watching TV, etc. It strengthens the lower back and stimulates the internal organs.

It is important to maintain the correct width between the feet, which is approximately equal to the width of the shoulder or width of the pelvis. When students unconsciously narrow the width between their feet, they will experience instability that often results in developing a bad habit of turning the back foot outward which will worsen the balance during the sitting back move.

After much practice, one should feel comfortable and agile in moving in and out of this position. At this point one is ready to do push hands. Both the "sit back" move and the "forward lean" move contribute to the up and down flow of internal energy and the qi in the body. Therefore, they are important components in the internal energy and qi circulation during the playing of Tai Chi Form.

When a sit back move is executed following the forward lean move, these steps occur:

- The back foot and core, with the compressed abdominal muscles, pull the body back with the heel of the front foot grabbing the ground to help control the backward movement.
- Maintaining parallel feet. If the back foot turns outward, the sitting position is not stable. One is easily pushed out of balance backwards (see Picture VI-5). When the body is facing the opponent and both feet are parallel, the ward off move will be effective on both sides of body (see Picture VI-7 & VI-8). If the back foot turns outward, then there is a strong side and a weak side where an opponent could take advantage. The situation gets even worse if one wants to take a step back. Now the outturned leg is dangerously exposed to be kneed by the opponent (see Picture VI-6). Equally problematic is taking a step forward with that outturned foot.
- When sitting back, try to sit deep enough that the tops of both upper legs are even to each other (see Picture IV-3) and one is facing the opponent squarely.

- When the sit back move reaches completion, the energized (compressed) abdominal muscle will keep the buttocks fully tucked in and also give the spine a slight upward stretch (not as much as the stretch of the forward lean move). This minor stretch does indicate that the weight of the upper body and the force from the sit back motion are now supported by the abdominal muscle and not the lower spine, an important consideration to maintain the health of the lower back.

- The sit back body posture will vary depending on the application. In the primary posture, the body is approximately perpendicular to ground with a crease of the body at the groin region (see Picture IV-5). This posture is useful to ward off and throw an opponent off balance when the opponent is attacking in the upper torso region. This posture is most common in the Form.

- Another posture is where the body leans back in the sitting position with the head, torso, and the forward leg forming a straight line leaning back (see Picture VI-9). This is to defend against an attack coming high. With this move, it is possible to partially lift the forward-stretched opponent off the ground, turn and throw him (see Picture VI-10, VI-11). In Tai Chi classics, this is described as "when he comes high at you, make him go higher". This move is practiced in the Form such as one of the moves in "Parting the Wild Horse's Mane".

- Another sitting posture is where the body leans forward toward ground in the sitting position (see Picture VI-12). This is to defend against an attack coming low. With this move, it is possible to drag down the opponent even lower to destabilize him and throw him (see Picture VI-13 & VI-14). In Tai Chi classics, this is described as "when he comes low at you, make him go lower". This move is practiced in the Form in moves such as "Turn Body Brush Knee Push Step".

Turn At the Waist and Stretch of the Spine

The benefits of stretching the spine during forward lean and sit back moves have been discussed above. With Internal Discipline, turning of the body is accomplished at the waist not at the "kua" or hip. Picture VI-15 & VI-16 show the turning move from waist in "Jade Lady Works at the Shuttle". It is important that the spine is stretched during this move to minimize the pressure on the discs in the spine so the rotation of the spine will not injure the discs. This is especially important when one tries a move as in Picture VI-11 in which one has to handle the additional weight of the opponent. In Classical Tai Chi, in almost every move, there is some consideration given to protect the health of the spine.

The Importance of Heel on the Ground

Tai Chi, unlike other martial arts, emphasizes a stance with heel on the ground. This could be explained both from a martial arts and health benefits viewpoint. Most other martial arts emphasize offensive movements and utilize a considerable amount of momentum force. When one is on the ball of his foot, it is easier to push off and rush the opponent and build momentum in the movement. When one depends on momentum in his strike force, it is not important that he is well connected with the ground. After all, a flying heavy object in the air could knock a person down. However, for the delivery of internal force, "fajin", a solid connection to the ground is very important. The power generated at the yin-yang junction is delivered against the supporting part (yin part) of the body, which in turn is supported by the ground through the heel. As I will demonstrate in the latter section, some of these fajin moves involve very small movements. The so-called one inch punch is an example of it. Now if the supporting structure has slack, flabbiness, or play in its various locations, an eighth of an inch here, a quarter inch there, the power reaching the opponent will dissipate to a small fraction of what was generated. So, not only does one have to be able to generate internal power, but also one has to be able to deliver it to the opponent with minimum loss. During fajin, if the heel is not on the ground, the reaction force from fajin will likely push the heel down until touching the ground. This slack in the body will diminish the power delivered.

Practicing of Tai Chi Form to achieve the maximum health benefits is to have internal energy continually circulating in the body without interruption, i.e. the circulating qi. To achieve this, every movement needs to generate certain internal energy in order to maintain the continuity. The firm contact of the heel with the ground, such as in "Brush Knee Push Step", or the pull of body backwards by the heel, such as in "Cloud Hand" and "Repulse Monkey", are important movements to generate internal energy in the body. Without the contribution from the heel to ground movements, there will be many breaks in the circulation of internal energy.

Another example showing the importance of heel on the ground is the move, "Rotate Body Punch". In Picture VI-17, I have just turned my body, aligned the back foot to the body, and am ready to sit back. In Picture VI-18, just when my back foot's heel touches the ground, I can feel a surge of energy moving from my core to the rising arm and at the same time, an energy surge down the leg to the ground. If the back foot and body alignment is missing, the back foot turned outward at an angle to the body, for example, not only will such power surge be diminished or nonexistent, but the hip and knee joints will feel uncomfortable or painful depending on the degree of the outturn of the foot. There are several heel-touch- ground situations in the Form where one could experience this effect. What I try to emphasize here is that the body structure or body alignment which can handle the energy of the reaction force to be absorbed by the ground efficiently is crucial. Any deficiency in that part of structure will result in inefficient fajin, discontinuity in the internal energy circulation, and potential of joint injuries.

Silk Reeling Exercise and Offline Exercise

One might define silk reeling exercises as a continuous symmetrical simple internal movement or movements. When it is done correctly, one will achieve a continuous energy flow in the body. It is a "neigong" exercise. The 108 move long Form in the hand of an advanced practitioner is a giant, complex silk reeling exercise with internal energy circulating continuously from beginning to the end of the Form. However, for less advanced students, it is best to start with a few simple moves converting to a continuous symmetrical exercise to practice. With that, one will be able to learn gradually how to move with internal discipline and enjoy the sensation of internal energy circulation. Many movements in the Long Form can be extracted and converted into silk reeling exercise. For beginning students, we often start them on the Body Turning move and an exercise alternately raising right and left arm from hanging down position to the waist high position and then lower them to complete the cycle. The Turning Move is the easiest to teach and to be appreciated. The raising arm silk reeling exercise looks extremely simple, but is a challenge to achieve as an internal move. More advanced students enjoy the walking silk reeling exercise and also the exercise derived from "Cloud Hands". The walking exercise emphasizes the stimulation of the intestine and other organs in the abdominal cavity, while the Cloud Hands exercise emphasizes the stimulation of muscles, tendons, and blood flow along the spine and the back. Those who have practiced these exercises regularly all experience a sense of rejuvenation and improved well being. These exercises offer a quick way to enjoy the sensation of internal movements and energy circulation.

Students are encouraged to practice simple internal moves whenever there is spare time in their daily life such as waiting at a copier, walking in the supermarket, riding in the car, and etc. This is called offline practice. The advantage of this is not only to have more time to practice, but also to get used to the idea of incorporating internal moves into everyday life. The other advantage is that such offline exercise is carried out in a casual and relaxed mood with more of a chance to let subconscious play a part. The objective is to learn internal moves piecemeal and then integrate them into the Form play.

Integration of Internal Discipline into Form Play

One could learn internal moves piecemeal then integrate them into Form play. However, there are such numerous movements in the 108 Long Form, how can this be taught or learned? Besides, since it is moving continuously, one has to achieve "internal" at any moment, any location in the Form, not just those obvious moves, so that continuity of the energy circulation can be achieved. Examining my own experience, I learned by the old way, many years of practice, following my teacher's instruction faithfully. The majority of students nowadays are less patient than in the old times and much more anxious regarding results. The teacher needs to be able to explain the common principles behind the moves so that the students can progress faster. After much progress in introducing the fundamentals of Internal Discipline to students, students still have considerable difficulties in carrying out certain internal moves. I finally realized that the problem is in establishing engagement between the arm and the internal core so that they became a single unit in motion and that internal energy could be delivered through the arm to the hand without degradation. This engagement certainly can be achieved successfully in the old way with years of practice. But, success also depends highly on the aptitude of the person. Many people may never get it no matter how long they have practiced.

In my search for a teaching method, which can provide more dependable results, by analyzing my own movements, I found out the answer is surprisingly simple. The following is a post on the Forum for distance learning students:

HOW TO MOVE THE ARM AND THE CORE BODY AS A UNIT

We have spent considerable time on the topic of learning internal discipline and how to apply it in the Tai Chi movements. I realize many of you are still have difficulties in this area. I have been examining my own movements and trying to come up with a better way of teaching this. I think I have found an approach which can accelerate the learning curve. I have tested it out on my students in class, and it seems to work well. I want to share this with you.

Some of you may already practice what I am going to talk about. After all, you will develop this naturally by just practicing what I have shown in the video. My desire to shorten the learning curve might have been viewed with disapproving eye by the old Masters of the past. They believe in diligent practice and self discovery: not hand held by their teacher. I hope I am not doing Mencius' story about a farmer who was impatient watching his seedlings grow so slowly that he went to the field and pulled the seedlings up to help their growth!

In the beginning of the learning process, you are instructed to relax or forget about the shoulder and the arm, just concentrate on the abdomen and the back for the internal movements. This is to eliminate the common habit of moving from the arm or shoulder. The shoulder and arm just follow the movements from the internal core. For most people, the difficulty here is to find the neural pathways in the core which can make the internal move you intended.

After you practice the form in this way for a while you will develop some knack for moving from the core. Then comes the second stage of learning which is to integrate your arm with the internal movements and to expand the circulating internal energy and qi from the torso to the arm, the palm and the finger tips. Previously, I talked about the incorporation of "Yi", or martial art intent, in the movement. With practice, one will achieve the state where the arm and the internal core move as "One" and, that the internal energy and qi flow with the "Yi" of the movements to the palm and the finger tips.

By examining my own movements I found that, in this state, my arm or elbow constantly exerts a slight downward stretch or pull on the shoulder. This stretch firmly engages the arm to the shoulder. Since the elbow is always lower than the shoulder, there is a downward stretching force causing the shoulder to sink which in turn connects it to the core enabling the arm and the core to move as "One". The stretching force involved here is quite subtle and small, just sufficient to achieve the engagement. Those who have already achieved such engagement in practice probably don't even know it. One can sense the difference if one purposely left out the stretch.

Additionally, between the arm, shoulder and core, it is often difficult to tell which part is leading or following. It is best to always keep the shoulder passive as a follower. But the arm, or the finger, especially the elbow, filled with "yi", may sometimes give the sensation of leading the movement. The synergistic effects between core movements and the engagement of the arm and core give unexpected results. When I try engagement exercises on students new to my class, it seems to help them learn how to make the core move. This is an unexpected and extremely significant benefit. What it means is that a person, not knowing how to move the internal core muscle, after learning how to engage the arm with the core, can use the arm to train the movement of the core muscle. I did not expect this, but after further thought, I realized that if one can engage the arm and core truly as an integral unit, then it is natural that either arm or the core can lead the movement. Once the core muscle is trained, then it can lead the movement with internal power. With this capability one can then use the arm movement to train all the movements in the Form, even the most obscure transition moves, to be internal and achieve the goal of internal energy circulating without break when playing the Form. Applying this method, I find that the training of internal movement and engagement with the core can be greatly accelerated.

The discussion here is concentrated on the relationship between core and arm, not core and other parts of the body, because none are as difficult as the arm. Leg movements, as well as the folding movement around the spine, are well trained in the Square Form. Arm movements have been the most difficult and are left for the Round Form.

Early in my training with Master Young, he cited the three "no" rules when playing the Form:

1. Knee does not project beyond the toe
2. Elbow does not go beyond the back
3. Hand does not go over the head.

The first rule has been discussed before. One of the considerations regarding the second rule is that if one hits the opponent behind them by thrusting the elbow behind one's back, the chest will be fully expanded. There is no give in the chest to absorb the reaction force bouncing back from the hit. It will shock the heart which is bad for the health. There are not many occasions when one needs to raise the hand over their head during martial art applications. In addition, one will leave a large opening exposing the body for attack when the hand goes over the head. In view of the discussion on arm-core engagement, if the hand is over the head, very little engagement can be accomplished. The hand is isolated and weak. Therefore, in Classical Tai Chi the hand is always lower than the head. As a result, the elbow is always lower than the shoulder. The elbow is always in a position to stretch the shoulder down to achieve engagement throughout the Form.

Tight-Compact Form

So far, the discussions are centered on Mid-Compact Form. That is the focus of my teaching program. The Tight-Compact Form has the same characteristics as Mid-Compact with small differences in its emphasis. It is quite easy and almost a natural progression for an advanced Mid-Compact practitioner to learn the Tight-Compact.

Certainly one of the major distinctions is its small step size (see Picture IV-2). It would be difficult for an opponent to tell which foot is weight bearing and which foot is free to move. In fact, shifts from one to the other are now instant and effortless. The larger the step size, the slower and more obvious are the foot movements. The progression from Large Frame to Tight-Compact Frame may be considered as "from Form to approaching Formless".

The upper body movements are more tightly coiled. Picture VI-20 to VI-23 show the "Brush Knee Push Step" moves in Mid-Compact Form while Picture VI-24 to VI-27 shows the same moves in Tight-Compact Form. In Picture VI-25 & VI-26, the tight coiling of the left arm, and in Picture VI-27, the elbow of the forward push arm moves toward the center of the body. All these differences give a stronger connection to the core and more intense internal energy and qi development than the Mid-Compact Form. All the moves are now pulled closer to the body and therefore sometimes it is called Small Circle Form. The Form can be practiced very fast, 2-3 minutes for the entire 108 Long Form. It is a necessary training for martial art applications. One can imagine when two expert Tai Chi masters are facing each other, they will probe each other with quick small movements. Every movement has its strength and weakness. If the movement is large, halfway through, the opponent will figure out how to take advantage of it. Large movements are useful only when the opponent is already out of balance, then one can use it to take down the opponent.

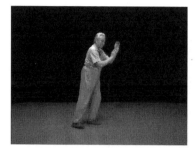 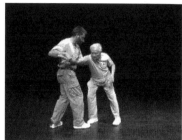

(Picture VI-1 and Picture VI-2)

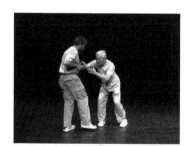 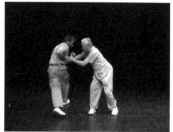

(Picture VI-3 and Picture VI-4)

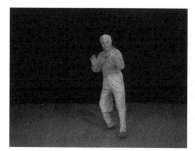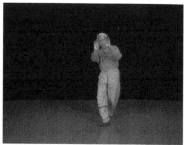

(Picture VI-5 and Picture VI-6)

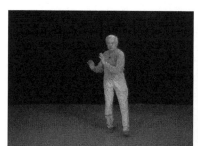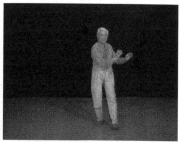

(Picture VI-7 and Picture VI-8)

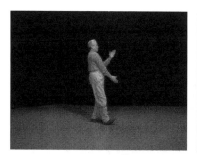 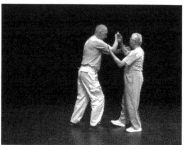

(Picture VI-9 and Picture VI-10)

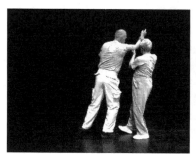 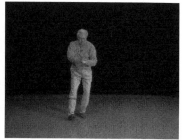

(Picture VI-11 and Picture VI-12)

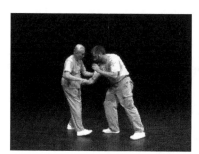 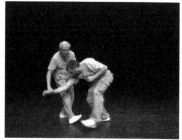

(Picture VI-13 and Picture VI-14)

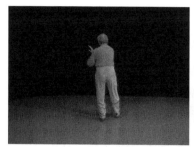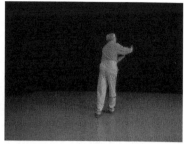

(Picture VI-15 and Picture VI-16)

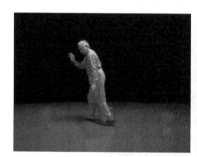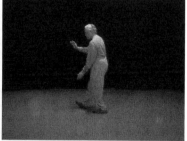

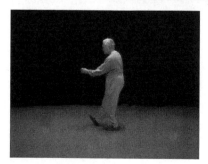

(Picture VI-17, Picture VI-18, Picture VI-19)

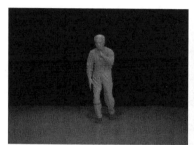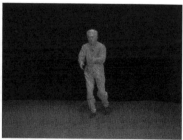

(Picture VI-20 and Picture VI-21)

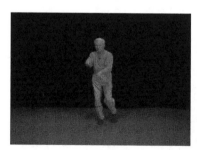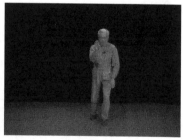

(Picture VI-22 and Picture VI-23)

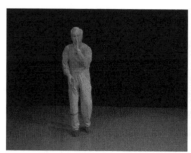 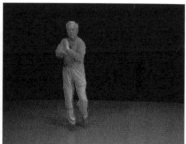

(Picture VI-24 and Picture VI-25)

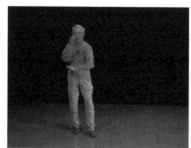 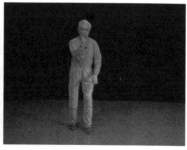

(Picture VI-26 and Picture VI-27)

CHAPTER VII:

RELAXING AND ENERGIZING

The topic of "energized" and "relaxed" has been touched upon before. A relaxed body and mind is the most commonly cited benefit of Tai Chi. Students spend countless hours trying to relax their shoulder, arm, face, breathing, etc. Therefore, the word "tension" is abhorred. The word "energized" used here is partly to avoid this stigma and partly to indicate that there is an active, transforming muscle tension for a specific purpose. The energy generated from this tension is called "jin" in Chinese. When an advanced practitioner plays the Form, there is a streak of active, transforming muscle tension circulating, zigzagging in an otherwise relaxed body giving rise to the sensation of stretching and energy flow. Fajin is a quick discharge of energy powered by a sudden tension in the core and delivered through the tightly coupled extremity. Muscle tension is a crucial part of Tai Chi. Much of our effort in practicing is trying to learn how to manage the differentiation between "energized" and "relaxed", or "yin" and "yang", in the body so that we can generate the energy we desire efficiently. On the other hand, nervous tension has to be absolutely eliminated in Tai Chi.

Several of my beginning students complain that when they sit back, their abdominal muscles are already tensed up for the pulling back movement. They are not able to, at the same time, turn the body at the waist to carry out the ward off move and draw the opponent off balance. One has to understand that energizing the "dantien" for certain move is different from tensing up the "dantien". Tensing or stiffening the dantien immobilizes the entire section of that part of the body indiscriminately. Energizing is a selective utilization of certain muscles for certain functions. Energizing has the character of agility, a sudden surge and ebb and is not static. Even the "tuck in" should be fluid in nature. So, even if one is fully tucked in, one should still have the feeling of suppleness ("soong" in Chinese) at the dantien to be able to carry out the body turning move or the ward off move using the waist.

A picture of what is going on during the sit back and ward off move mentioned above could be as follows: The tuck in move uses the Rectus Abdominus muscle, while the turning move uses the External and Internal Obliques. Even though both muscles are next to each other in the same region, with the yin-yang training in tai chi, one should be able to use its distinctive features independent of each other or in cooperation with each other. All those attributes mentioned above can be developed by practicing the Tai Chi Form. I have seen this among my students how they progress. They work off mental tension which will cause indiscriminate tenseness of the muscle and sharpen the yin-yang differentiation in the movement so that only the necessary muscle is energized while the rest of the body is relaxed.

There is a simple example one could try to experience this effect without much practice. The following is a discussion in our Forum.

Jim D. writes:

...... I understand the utility of redirecting incoming force, but when blocking, how is it that the arm remains soft and subtle (in order that we may listen), and not rigid as in external martial arts?

Master Hwa's response:

In the Forum 10, I discussed a similar question regarding the dantien where you need to be energized and yet not rigid. In short, the rigidity in external martial art is in-discriminatory with every muscle in the arm stiffened up to the maximum. In tai chi, only the necessary energizing is employed. In addition, your blocking of the opponent's arm should use a force just enough to ward off his arm. If you use too much force then it's no longer redirect, but push back, and you lost the advantage of redirect.

Therefore your ward-off move is very fluid and delicate. This can only be achieved when you are not stiff or rigid.

I have an experiment I want you to try: Try to press the back of your hand against say a door frame, just like you are blocking an opponent's incoming arm. Do you find that one side of your forearm muscle is energized while the other side, the muscle is relaxed? Let me know your results.

Jim D. responds:

I tried your suggestion to "press the back of your hand against say a door frame" several times and had several different experiences. They are as follows: (1) a tightening of the outside of my forearm and back arm, or (2) a tightening of the whole arm to include the fore arm and biceps and back arm, and (3) resistance from the door jamb which seemed to force me backwards as I pushed forward. These experiences seemed to be effected by the amount of pressure I applied.

Master Hwa's response:

Your experiments showed three different cases, illustrating some very interesting points:

1. This is the expected case. You should be able to block using only the outside muscle of the fore arm (extensor) while inside muscle of the fore arm (flexor and palmaris) should be completely

relaxed, in other words you only use the necessary muscle to achieve the task. Your arm is still supple and responsive and you can make counter move with the arm very quickly.

2. Here you are tensing or stiffening your entire arm, the muscles in the arm are stiffening indiscriminately. The arm has a wooden feeling and does not respond very quickly. One could achieve this state very easily by clenching the fist. That is why Classical Tai Chi has no clenched fist in its form.

3. Here you are applying a force beyond what your body structure (rooting) could support, just like forward fajin with the body perpendicular to the ground. When we apply a force there is an equal and opposite reaction force which needs to be absorbed by the ground through the body. If your body structure is not firmly supported by the ground in comparison to that of your opponent, in this case the door frame, your body will move when the force you apply is beyond what your body structure could support. That is why I emphasized in the Overview Video that fajin is useful only when you detect an opening in an opponent's movement, such as taking advantage of his body's momentum or deficiency in his rooting and striking without any forewarning. It is not a move with brutal force but with fineness

and sensitivity. That is the reason why training a Tai Chi fighter is much more difficult than training an external martial arts fighter.

I believe that case 1 is the natural response. Case 2 is a learned habit-a bad habit at that. Nowadays, all TV and movies show martial arts with tight fists and muscles bulging on the entire arm. People get brainwashed thinking this is the norm. This is purely for show. It would be a huge mistake if to think this is the way to fight. Practicing Tai Chi will refine the natural ability of using only the right muscle and the right amount of force in the movements and not affected by emotions such as fear or tenseness since the moves are now instinctive.

CHAPTER VIII:

IMPORTANT CONSIDERATIONS DURING FORM PLAYING

There are quite a few such considerations mentioned in almost every Tai Chi book. Here I select those which are not often mentioned or controversial to discuss below:

Form Playing Speed

The Square Form: Each movement in the Square Form always starts and ends with a complete stop. The movement itself is rather resolute and brisk. The playtime of the entire Form therefore consists of stopping time and movement time with both times comparable. The playtime I use is 14-15 min. It is better for a beginner to go a little slower, 16-20 min., to make certain that the student does not skip over the "stop" between the movements and to provide some thinking time. Speed of play in the Square Form is primarily for the consideration of learning and practice unlike that of the Round Form where more complex considerations must be taken into account.

The Round Form: In my video, the Round Form is played in the speed range from 8-12 minutes for the 108. This is a good speed range for daily practice of the Form for all levels. For the beginner, it is preferable to stay in the slower part of the range. In this way, students have more time to incorporate some internal into the movements. For advanced practitioners, one should also experience playing the form at slower and faster speeds.

Slower speeds: When the playing speed slows, the level of internal force of the movement does not change. In other words, if you stop your internal movement in the midway, you will find that the internal force remains energized (it is almost like an isometric exercise). So playing at slow speed gives you more time to sense and experiment with the details of the internal move. What is changing with slower speed is the slower circulation of the internal energy in the body. Eventually, one will have a diminished sense of circulating energy or energy flow becoming intermittent. That means the playing speed is too slow, which will probably happen when it is close to 20 minutes for the complete set.

Faster speeds: How fast one can play the form is limited by the internal energy possessed by the practitioner. Losing firm control of the movement, skipping details of the internal movement, building up tension and not being able to maintain the yin-yang differentiation are some of the signs that the playing speed is beyond the capability of the practitioner. When the speed reaches 4 minutes, Tight-Compact Form will be the natural choice. It is an exhilarating experience to play the 108 Long Form in the 2-3 min. range while maintaining the relax-energizing differentiation (yin-yang separation) in the body just as playing at the normal speed, and enjoying the rapid circulation of the internal energy. To achieve poise and relaxation at this speed is an important preparation for martial art application.

One does not learn to play this fast by practicing fast. The foundation is built at the regular speed where every detail is honed to perfection and where internal energy is developed to a high degree. In other words, one has to become robust internally before one tries to go fast.

Breathing

Breathing should be relaxed and natural with the mouth closed and tongue lightly touching the upper palate. The mouth should stay relaxed so that one can expel air through mouth if need to be, as during martial art applications. Some schools advise that students breath in or out following each movement's to and fro. In the Compact Form, the movements have lots of circular motions. One would have difficulty deciding at what point one should be breathing in or out. One should not add this undue burden and additional tension to the mind which is already overwhelmed in the early stages of learning. When one plays the Form fast as discussed above, one would have to go into hyperventilation, if he had to breathe in or out according to the to and fro of each movement. One should not try to incorporate breathing qi gong into Tai Chi. After all Classical Tai Chi its self is a much better motion induced qi gong than breathing qi gong.

Gaze During Tai Chi

In external martial arts, one is supposed to have a focused and stern gaze on the opponent. Tai Chi is just the opposite. It asks for a relaxed gaze with eyelid half open. When one focuses one's gaze on the opponent, other senses, such as touch, peripheral vision, and intuitive feel about the opponent's intent, suffers. Perhaps the most effective way to relax one's mind is first trying to relax the eye. When the eye is relaxed, the mind is relaxed and more receptive to broad sensory input and faster intuitive response.

Old masters, who were martial art purists, did not look favorably on practicing the Form with eyes closed. After all, they tried not to close the eye, even to avoid blinking. But for the non-martial art purist, trying to play the Form with eyes closed is an interesting test and useful training of nerve communication and muscular response between the feet and the rest of the body to keep balance and steadiness of the body. When one can do this without a balancing problem,   meditation in motion can be enhanced. I myself do try this from time to time.

Hands Touching

During the playing of Compact Round Form, one is truly meditation in motion with the body filled with qi. If accidently one's hands touch each other or other parts of the body, one will feel a shock and break the continuity of the circulation of energy and qi. There is no such restriction when playing Large Frame and Square Form since there is no such circulation in the body.

Indoor or Outdoor

Many of my distance learning students ask me about practicing outdoors. It is fine to do that with Large Frame and Square Form, or during the early learning stage. But, for the same kind consideration discussed above, it is best to play the Compact Round Form indoors for the advanced practitioner. A sudden gust of wind or stepping on a stone can shock and break the continuity of the circulation.

It seems contradictory that Tai Chi is a martial art and yet the Compact Round Form is played with such care and delicacy. That just shows the ingeniousness on the part of the old Masters developing this art with such a dual personality. It is a tool for combat but it is also a meditation for inner cultivation.

What to Wear in Class

When teaching Internal Discipline, the teacher needs to show the students how the core muscles move. Such a visual impression in students' mind will provide a guide for students to work toward it gradually. The teacher also needs to see student's movement in order to give any guidance. So, the clothing to wear in class has to be able to show the core movements as clear as possible. Those so-called "Tai Chi suit" hanging very loosely on the body are not suitable for this kind of class. Form-fitting shirts would be the preferable wear for Classical Tai Chi.

The Left Hand Form

The movements in the 108 Long Form are mostly non- symmetrical in regard to the right and left side of the body. We generally call the normal Form the "right hand Form". It is purely a name-not necessarily meaning that the right side of body is more emphasized. Because of the nonsymmetrical nature of the Form, It results in unbalanced development of the body when one practices this way day in and day out.

When one can play the right hand Form with ease, it is time to teach oneself to play the mirror image of the Form, so called "left hand Form". It is a very beneficial exercise. One can gain considerable insight into ones' Form playing. Students who have gone through this exercise have reported that they sense the weakness on the left hand Form initially indicating that they have already built up robustness on the right side. Eventually, when one plays the Form, one should alternate between right and left Form to insure balanced development.

CHAPTER IX:

TAI CHI FORM & DELIVERY OF POWER (FAJIN)

Training For Fajin

The power source behind Tai Chi moves has not been discussed very much in previous Tai Chi writings. One early description often used by most current writings is, "Jin(force) should be rooted in the feet, generated from the legs, controlled by the waist, and manifested through the fingers". This statement may be applicable to certain Large Frame moves which use the leg to generate the pushing force. But, it is not applicable in the Compact Form which generates power from the torso. The force transmitted through the leg is the reaction force from the waist which is absorbed by the ground. Much of the body structure of the yin part of the body takes this into consideration, such as the forward lean and sitting back body structure.

For those uninitiated, the question is always, how can such a soft, slow moving Tai Chi Form be preparation for martial arts? People admire the fast moving, full force punching and kicking motion in the Kata (Form) of external martial arts and consider that the only way to practice for delivering power. That was my thought, too, when I started to learn Tai Chi as a complete novice. My teacher, Young Wabu, always considered that unless the student was versed in the fundamentals (the Form), there was no point to teach the student applications. When I was starting, I was a forty year old with bad back, not very concerned about applications. My exposure to applications was primarily his demonstration of certain applications to illustrate the meaning of Form movements and learning the technique of push hands. And, occasionally, my teacher's daughter, Master Sonia Young would teach the students applications. She loved martial art applications even as a little girl and became a student of Wu Kung Yi in his famed Hong Kong Chien Chuan T'ai Chi Ch'uan Academy at age of eleven, practicing with his grown-up students on applications. I could see the exceptional power of my teachers and realized the power in Tai Chi. But, without mastering Internal Discipline, my movements were full of tension and used external force constantly. By the way, my back problem completely disappeared when I was learning Square Form. And, Round Form greatly strengthened my back.

For many years, I was working away from Rochester, NY, where my teacher was located. Luckily, I could remember his teaching very well allowing me to continue and improve my Form by myself. When I had achieved the level where internal energy circulated during Form practice and Form practice was completely subconscious, I discover that I could do fajin without consciously knowing that I was practicing fajin.

It is amazing that Masters of the past could have such insight that slow and seemingly soft movements could be an ideal tool to train a person to deliver exceptional power. What they discovered was that the slow movements with Internal Discipline trained a person in every little detail of that fajin move. After a person repeated the moves a thousand times, it becomes part of him and is available to use any moment he wishes at any power level or speed.

The full speed and power punch and kick of the Kata or Form of external martial arts, on the surface, seems a logical way to train. But, in fact, it has deficiencies. When a full speed punch or kick reaches its end point, the momentum of the movement has to be absorbed by the shoulder or hip joint to stop the movement which could cause hyperextension of the tendon in that joint. Since I am teaching Tai Chi in a Karate school, I hear stories about young and promising black belts who need to have their shoulder or hip repaired. Another subtle effect is that the intent of retraction at the end point (pull the punch) may carry over to actual applications which will result in shallow penetration of the power delivered. Some Karate students commented that Tai Chi fajin force seems to penetrate through the body, not just be concentrated at the point of impact, as they experienced in Karate.

The delivery of power during fajin may vary from an extended time delivery, such as in "Grasp Peacock's Tail" and "Jade Lady Works at the Shuttle".

The more interesting types of fajin are those that are delivered in a very short burst, where the receiver will feel jolted, shocked, like a concussion. In external martial arts, this effect is achieved by initiating the punch at a distance. When it lands on the receiver, all the force and momentum accumulated in the punch is delivered at once. But, in the case of Tai Chi fajin, the hand can already be in contact with the receiver, such as in 'stick to the opponent', when the power is delivered. Therefore, the sudden burst of power has to be generated purely from the internal source. Force generated from external limbs such as arms and legs have much longer duration and cannot be compacted into such a short burst. In fact, within internal moves, it is the upper quarter body movements that are most suitable to generate fajin with explosive force, i.e. from relaxing to peak power in an instant. Two examples are discussed below:

Examples of Fajin
One-Inch-Punch

This term was made famous by Bruce Lee. In Tai Chi Classics on Thirteen Postures, this move can be classified as Peng (push). In the Pictures IX-1, IX-2, & IX-3, I demonstrate this move on Tom by placing a loosely held fist against the protective pad on Tom. At the same time, I ask Jim to touch my arm to feel the response of the muscle in the arm to such move. This was the first time that either Jim or Tom experienced this move. Jim reported that the arm was completely relaxed. When the move was initiated, the arm suddenly felt rigid and quickly relaxed again. During that momentary stiffness of the arm, the internal power passed through the arm and delivered to the opponent. It is essential to have a relaxed arm prior to the punch to get the maximum effect. Even placing too much intent on that move may reduce its power because excess intent will introduce tension into the arm prior to move. In other words, one has to do the move primarily subconsciously with minimum intent. The use of a loosely held fist is for the same reason of maintaining a relaxed arm. When the internal power surges out of the core, just tighten the fist to stiffen the arm and deliver the power. My seventeen year old student, Ike, made a very astute observation that the sudden stiffening of the fist and the arm started just when the surge of power reached the opponent. The stiffening is a natural response to the feedback of a sensation of resistance. The stiffened arm, then, delivers the bulk of the power to the opponent. If the stiffening occurs before the surge, the power will be reduced. The whole process may last only a fraction of a second. Yet, practicing the Form trains one to accomplish this subconsciously.

The body structure shown in the pictures is worthy of discussion here. Tom is in the forward lean posture in preparation for incoming force. For the person delivering the punch, there is an equal and opposite reaction force returning to that person. To handle that reaction force, I have to have a body structure better than the receiver. In this case, my body structure is not good for a forward fajin. The reaction force will push me back instead of Tom. What makes this punch work as shown in the pictures is that the punch has a major component of an uplifting force. It lifted Tom's body partially off the ground. Then, the minor forward force knocked Tom backwards. The reaction force from the uplifting force is a downward force started at the waist, down the leg and absorbed by the ground. In this case, my upright posture has the advantage. The stance I am using here is actually Tight-Compact Form. In all the pictures shown in this book, the stance I use for fajin are all Compact stance. It just illustrates that one does not need a large stance to generate power, as most people think. In fact, Compact Form has the advantage that one can easily optimize one's posture for fajin in response to changing situations.

Tom was protected from internal injury with a four-inch foam pad. The presence of the pad neutralized an important characteristic of fajin , i.e. the explosive nature of the force. Once, I was demonstrating this punch to a group of Tai Chi aficionados. One of the participants was an amateur boxer in his younger days, very familiar with the body punch. He insisted on trying this on him without the pad. I reluctantly agreed to try on him with a punch of reduced power. Yet, the effect was more dramatic. He just collapsed backwards toward the ground. Luckily, people stood next to him on both sides and were able to grab him before he hit the ground. The sudden impulse of the punch was too fast for him to readjust his body to neutralize the power, as Tom did.

The punches in the Compact Form as shown in Picture IX-4 (beginning of the punch) and Picture IX-5 (end of the Punch) are identical to the one-inch punch in the demonstration. The fist is a hollow fist with pointed knuckles, not tightly held. It is designed to strike at an opponent's mid-body, a soft part of the body. If the punch intended to hit a bony part of the body, such as the chin, it would hurt the fist. That would violate the rule that every move in Tai Chi should be good for both health and martial art applications. In the Large Frame Form, the punch often fully stretches to the shoulder-high position.

Cai (yank or jerk)

Cai is another move in the Thirteen Postures. The following is an example of the application of Cai and an illustration of how the power of the move is generated. In Picture IX-6, I have blocked and held Tom's arm. Picture IX-7, Tom tries to kick me. Just as he initiated the kick, I detected his intent and already engaged my core to Cai (yank) him. In this case, the Cai move is intended to draw Tom forward and sideways so that he will not ram into me. The initial power of Cai to destabilize Tom is shown in Pictures IX-10 & IX-11.

This Cai move has the same characteristics as the punch move discussed above. The power reaches its peak instantly from a relaxed start. My arm is blocking Tom's and is both energized and relaxed (see discussion in Chapter VII). The power is delivered instantly, mostly subconsciously, once his intention is detected. This is also an example of what Tai Chi Classics' say "When opponent does not move, I do not move. When he plans to move on me, I get to him first"

In the Form, there are several different moves to practice the Cai move some of which have slightly different applications. Practicing the move shown in Picture IX-10 & IX-11, is in the kicking section of the Form, see Picture IX-12 & IX-13. The hand movements in the pictures practice the Cai move while the foot movements practice the kicking routine. Many of the movements in the Form are designed this way. In other words, one limb practices a move for one purpose, while the others practice for some other purposes. This is a very economical design, packing much practice opportunity into the 108 Long Form. Another such example is the "Brush Knee Push Step". One hand is forward fajin while the other hand is a ward-off move, warding off an attack coming at the abdominal region (see Picture VI 22 & VI 23). During applications, each move will likely apply by itself not together as in the Form.

Paradoxically and contrary to common belief, practicing the seemingly soft and gentle Compact Form Classical Tai Chi develops internal energy and power while practicing the martial art of push hands and sparring should develop sensitivity and finesse.

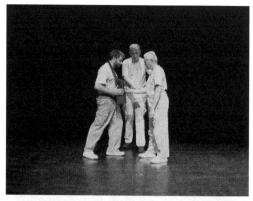

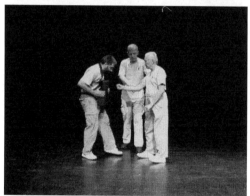

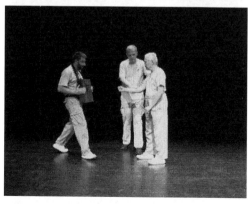

(Picture IX-1, Picture IX-2, Picture IX-3)

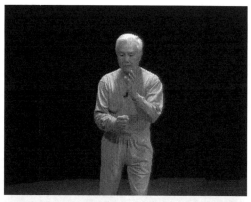

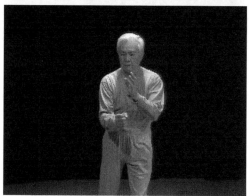

(Picture IX-4 and Picture IX-5)

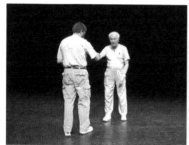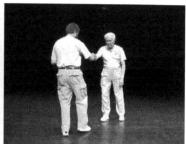

(Picture IX-6 and Picture IX-7)

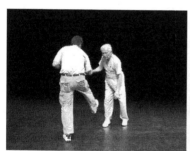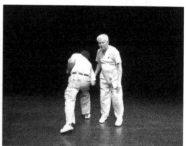

(Picture IX-8 and Picture IX-9)

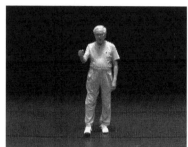
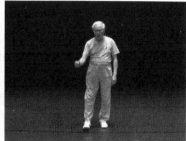

(Picture IX-10 and Picture IX-11)

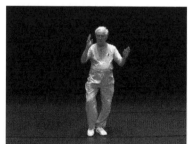
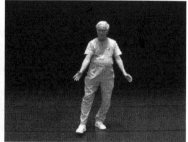

(Picture IX-12 and Picture IX-13)

CHAPTER X:

A LOOK AT THE LOGICAL
STRUCTURE OF TAI CHI

I have so far discussed many topics in Classical Tai Chi and also certain interconnections between these topics. Here I will try to pull together as much of these interconnections to peer into the logical structure built up by the early Tai Chi Masters. I am certain there are more advanced topics which I have omitted in this book. I believe what we have here covers the basic building blocks of Tai Chi to show at least what its foundation looks like. I am especially interested in how Tai Chi Form is designed to be useful for martial art applications and also good for health and how early Tai Chi Masters could structure the Form to achieve these two goals simultaneously.

Certainly one of the major foundation blocks is the definition of internal move -"Every movement in Tai Chi Form has to have two complementary parts of the body, a moving part (called the yang part) and a stationary part (called the yin part). When the yin-yang junction is located in the torso of the body, it is an internal move. When it is outside of the torso it is an external move." This definition has huge implications on Tai Chi martial arts applications as well as its health benefits. From the health benefits viewpoint, movements using internal discipline penetrate to the deep recesses of the torso, stimulating and invigorating the organs and the circulatory system.. The body further benefits from the circulating internal energy and qi during Form playing. These are the primary reasons why Tai Chi enhances the robustness of the body's internal systems.

From a martial art viewpoint, in addition to the fact that internal power generated based on this definition is the primary power source for Tai Chi, the requirement to have yin part of the body during movement means one cannot jump attack since that will result in all yang, no yin. That means Tai Chi is basically a defensive martial art. All the strategy, tactics and movements are developed based on a defensive posture, waiting until the opponent attacks, neutralizing the attack, and finding an opening to counter the attack.

Instead of pushing back at the opponent's attack, the best known defensive strategy of Tai Chi is to follow and stick to the opponents' move, neutralize or drain off its power and then counterattack. In order to be able to follow and stick to the opponent, one has to be relaxed, sensitive and quick on the feet, matching the opponents move with ease and anticipation. That is one reason that the Compact Form optimizes body posture to achieve lightness and nimbleness through parallel feet, compact movements, and avoidance of "double heavy".

Tai Chi applications emphasize stickiness or adherence to the opponent. This is useful only because this complements the fajin move perfectly. The characteristics of Fajin are

- Delivery of Fajin is most effective when already in contact with the opponent such as sticking to the opponent.
- Delivery of fajin is most effective when the hand in contact with the opponent is sufficiently relaxed to allow "listening" or "tien jin"- the objective of sticking to the opponent.
- Fajin has the ability to go from relaxation to full power instantly. When one sticks to the opponent and detects a weakness in opponent's move, one can suddenly counter attack with fajin without telegraphing the intent. If the capability of fajin is not available, even when one detects weakness in the opponent, one will not be able to take full advantage of those fleeting opportunities.

Tai Chi Form practice uses a unique approach to develop internal energy and the power for martial arts applications such as fajin. This unique approach employs slow movements and retains the energy and power internally without projecting the power. This is completely opposite to other martial arts' training method. I have said previously that the advantage of slow motion allows one to practice the details of the move deliberately and thoroughly. By not projecting the power, one avoids injuries to the shoulders and avoids forming the habit of "pulling the punch". Fajin is known to pack a sudden burst of power which can shock the opponent. But, it also shocks the person who delivers the fajin. If one practices full power fajin on an imaginary opponent, a punching bag or dummy, the effect of jarring over time will have a detrimental effect on the heart and other internal organs. Training with the Tai Chi Form avoids all these pitfalls.

A common thread among the discussions in this book is the attention to the body structure or body alignment which is a major building block of the logical structure of Tai Chi.

Early Masters must have had an in-depth understanding of body mechanics and its impact on health and on the transmission and delivery of force. They meticulously built their understanding into every move in the Form. The rigorous and calculated approach they took is a worthy comparison to any scientific endeavor nowadays. The common thread in the emphasis on body mechanics is the concern about preserving and improving the health of the joints, such as those in the spine, hip, knee and ankle. When the joints are properly aligned in the body, there will not be any shear force or torque force in the joints to cause damage. At the same time, such a straight path structure is also ideal for transmitting force, energy and qi without any blockage or slack. Therefore it is also correct for martial art applications and qi gong.

Attention on the spine includes: protecting spine from excessive compression forces, giving the spine opportunity to stretch from time to time, strengthening the muscles and tendons around the spine through Form practice. Attention on the hip, knee, and ankle includes: avoiding overextension of the joints, such as the knee projecting beyond the toe and high kicks, avoiding torque or shear force in the ankle, knee, and hip joints by following rules such as "hand follows the foot, elbow follows the knee, and shoulder follows the hip" or "upper and lower body following each other".

I will use the following sequence of pictures of Cloud Hands in Mid-Compact Form to illustrate the various points made previously in this book. Cloud Hands involves constant body turning. Notice, in these turns, the movements follow the rule of "hand follows the foot, elbow follows the knee". There is no torque or twist within each side of the body, right side or left side. Each side of the body is geared for up and down energy flow without any hindrance. Each side of the body follows the yin-yang rule that one side is turning while the other side remains still. Therefore, two sides of the body fold and unfold using the spine as the hinge. Picture X-12 shows the back is open around the spine while Picture X-10 shows the folding of the back around the spine. Each side of the body shows extension (Picture X-4) and contraction (Picture X-5) alternately. The "arm swing up move" is an upper quarter body movement tightly coupled with the core. This move together with the heel pull move create intense internal movements and energy flow up and down that side of the body, which is more easily visible from the back, such as Picture X-11, X-12, X-13, & X-14.   These intensive movements center around the spine, strengthening the muscle and connective tissue and blood flow around the spine. It is a very beneficial movement for the spine. Whenever I demonstrate this sequence, everyone is surprised at the contrast between the front view, very relaxed and seemingly effortless, and the back view, intense muscle undulating motion in the torso.

Tai Chi is sometime described as "outside cotton, inside steel". This is a good example of it.

Poor posture may not matter to young people for a while. Eventually, the problem catches up as the person ages. When one can keep the joints healthy even at old ages while the Internal Discipline keeps the body's internal systems robust, it is truly "live forever in the spring season of the life".

The following examples illustrate the above.

Picture X-1 shows a Tai Chi posture very popular among Tai Chi practitioners now, but having lost much of the well thought out structural elements in an equivalent Classical Tai Chi posture, see Picture X-2.

The concave curvature in the lower back region in Picture X-1 indicates localized compression and stress concentration of the spine in the lower back region. The punch motion in the Form will create a reaction force adding more stress at that location. This situation will be substantially worse if the punch hits the opponent since the reaction force will be much higher. In fact, it may bend the body further backwards hurting the lower back and losing the power. A group of Tai Chi enthusiasts of this style in Shanghai practiced together regularly, including push hands and sparring. At old age, every one of them had lower back bone spur problems.

In Picture X-2, the spine and back leg form a straight line to allow the reaction force transmitted along the straight path to be absorbed by the ground, without any stress concentrated along the spine. In addition, the energized abdominal muscles exert an upward stretch force on the spine which serves to minimize the compression stress along the spine.

The back leg is crucial in this forward punch move, since most of the reaction force from the punch passes through the back foot to be absorbed by the ground. In Picture X-1, with the back foot turned outward, not in line with the body, there is a torque force and a shear force in the hip joint, knee joint, and ankle. These forces increase greatly if the move actually strikes an opponent. Such a shear force is detrimental to the connective tissue in the joints. The proper posture is shown in Picture X-2 in which the back leg is in line with the body, "hand follows the foot, elbow follows the knee". There is no twist in any of the joints, so the leg can take the reaction force without damage to the joints.

From a martial arts consideration, any of these structural deficiencies, a concave bend at the lower back or twists in any of the joints of the back, leg will cause the weakness or sagging under the pressure of the reaction force resulting in the diminishing power of the forward punch. In addition, with the out-turned back foot, the posture lacks mobility and is not the light and nimble move expected in Tai Chi. This posture is awkward to sit back on the out turned back foot. It is awkward to take a step back exposing the out-turned leg in the front. It is awkward to take a step forward, since the out-turned back foot has to loop around to move forward.

Attention to the health of the joints is especially important for the late starter, starting to learn Tai Chi as an adult as most of new students are today. They have much less tolerance to shear stress in their joints and cannot readily grow and strengthen their joints to unusual demands like a young kid can. In the Tai Chi world, there are many practitioners trained in their childhood as dancers and acrobats and convert to Tai Chi practitioners later. Their Tai Chi dance performances are entertaining and a delight to the audience in public demonstrations. Picture X-3 is an example of this. This is not something an adult should aspire to. After all, the real benefit of Tai Chi is the development of Internal Discipline in the body, not a fancy dance routine.

Notice the knee projecting beyond the toe and the twist at the ankle in this picture. I wonder how long she can keep on doing this.

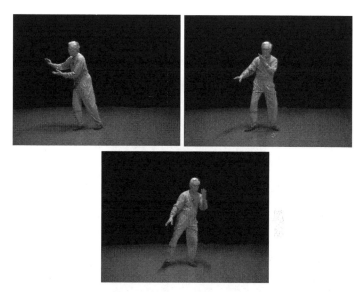

(Picture X-4, Picture X-5, Picture X-6)

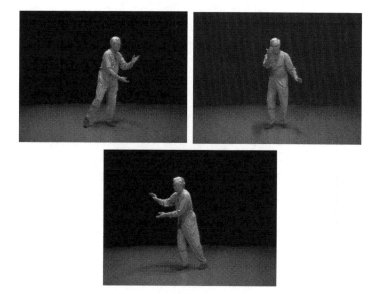

(Picture X-7, Picture X-8, Picture X-9)

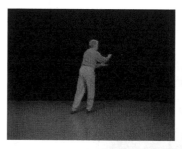
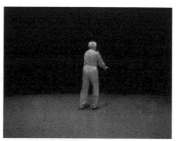
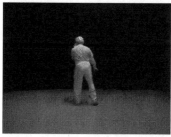

(Picture X-10, Picture X-11, Picture X-12)

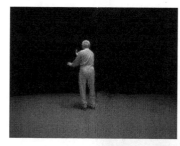
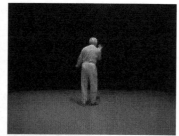
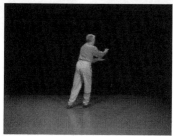

(Picture X-13, Picture X-14, Picture X-15)

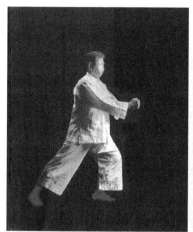
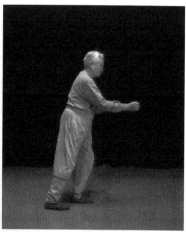
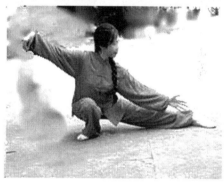

(Picture X-1, Picture X-2, Picture X-3)

CHAPTER XI:

TAI CHI & CHINESE PHILOSOPHY

Chinese philosophies are well known for their profound visions and eloquent ideas. They often appear to be abstract and distant from personal practical application. Yet, in Classical Tai Chi, these philosophies are applied systematically not just conceptually, but in actual physical applications where the practitioner can personally sense and appreciate the implications of these philosophical ideas. They will gain greatly both an appreciation of classical Chinese philosophies and Classical Tai Chi.

Tai Chi originated entirely in China, unlike martial arts which originated from the Shaolin Temple (so called Kung fu in the west) which is influenced by India's Buddhism. Even though the early history of Tai Chi is not well recorded, it is generally accepted that it evolved over many centuries to reach its present form. Therefore it embodies the most deep-seated spirit of Chinese philosophy with very unique characteristics as a martial art. This spirit is rooted in the I-Ching, but is elaborated and developed in major classics such as Lao-Tzu, Chuang -Tzu, Sun-Tzu, Meng-Tzu, etc.

Three of the books mentioned above, I-Ching , Lao-Tzu, and Chuang Tzu are also important philosophical foundations of Taoism. So, Tai Chi and Taoism share some of the same philosophical heritage. There is also the story about the mystical Taoist, Chang San- Feng who supposedly developed the early form of Tai Chi by observing fighting movements of animals. Certainly Tai Chi and Taoist religion both are known to esteem health and longevity. Buddhism, on the other hand, is ambivalent about health and longevity. Even though the original intent of Shaolin martial arts is for health and self-defense, the philosophy of Buddhism discourages undue attention on the human body, considering it to be a temporary abode for the soul and therefore not important. Some Buddhist's writings refer to human body as a "smelly leather bag". On the other hand, Tai Chi has the saying, "do not let a fly land on your shoulder", during martial arts application, meaning, treasure the body, take no punishment. The difference in such thinking reflects on the development of these two martial arts and in their way of training.

When early Tai Chi masters lectured their students, they often used quotes from these philosophical classics to make their points. As these classics were important text books in classical education during that period, students were familiar with these books and were taught to revere them for their teaching of the nature of things. Therefore using quotes from these books to explain Tai Chi's principles impressed students greatly. After the turn of the twentieth century, modern education replaced classical education. Students are not that familiar with these books any more. The use of these quotes in teaching Tai Chi has become much less prevalent.

I-Ching (The Book of Change)

This is the earliest known book in China with a known written version dated back to 1000 BC while the symbols representing yin – yang and eight trigrams were invented many thousand years before that. It is a very complex book with many different aspects including divination, cosmology, mathematics (binary number system), morals, and the philosophy of the nature of things.

For example, the eight directions used in Tai Chi is said to follow the orientation of the eight trigrams. Certainly the concept of yin and yang is the foundation of Tai Chi (as well as the foundation of Chinese medicine, biology etc).

Yin and Yang

Everything in the universe exists in an opposite and complementary pair, such as male and female, sun and moon, earth and heaven, fire and water, dominance and submission, soft and hard etc. Yin and yang constantly evolve or change from one to the other cyclically so that not one entity continually dominates the opposite entity for long. If the imbalance was persistant, it would lead to distress of the system. Since all entities evolve into its counterpart, every entity has within it the seeds of the counterpart.

Every aspect at every level in Tai Chi follows the principles of yin and yang. Here are some notable examples:

- Every movement in Tai Chi has yang (the moving part of body) and yin (the stationary part of body supporting the moving part and providing majority of the power). This requirement minimizes any movement involving the entire body moving with a momentum, such as jump off attack- a common move in external martial arts. Each Form movement is often a combination of several sets of yin-yang pairs in motion simultaneously. However the primary pair of yin-yang of that movement is always located in the torso.

- When practicing the Tai Chi Form, certain portion of the body is completely relaxed while other parts of the body are energized by the internal movements. "Relaxing" and "energizing" is therefore constantly maintained and evolved in the body. If the body is mostly relaxed without energizing from the internal movement, then it is too much yin, not enough yang to balance it. On the other hand, external martial arts usually tense up the entire body. Then, it is all yang and no yin.

- We play the Form slowly with the intent of developing instinctive swift response during martial art applications. "Slow" grows the seed of "swift". "Swift" retains the character of "tranquil".

- Softness and yielding concealed the hidden potential of "fajin (sudden burst of power)". During "fajin", one does not need to fully commit his body so that "fajin" and "yielding" could proceed in cycles.

- Round Form and Square Form outwardly could not be more diametrically opposite to each other. Yet, in the Square Form, there are seeds of Round Form and in the Round Form, there is hidden Square Form.

Lao-Tzu Tao Te Ching

Lao-Tzu was said to be written around 500 B. C. More commonly it is known as Tao Te Ching. It is a book of small size, but exerts great influence. I shall quote certain relevant passages directly from the book for discussion and demonstration:

Lao-Tzu Te-Tao Ching

Robert G. Hendricks, Ballantine Books, New York, 1989

Translation based on a newly discovered manuscript buried 168 B. C.

Page 47

When people are born, they're supple and soft;

When they die, they end up stretched out firm and rigid;

Therefore we say that the firm and rigid are companions of death,

While the supple, the soft, the weak, and the delicate are companions of life.

Note: Practicing Tai Chi is to get rid of rigidity and achieve suppleness.

Page 12

The softest, most pliable thing in the world runs roughshod over the firmest thing in the world.

Page 49

In the whole world, nothing is softer and weaker than water.

And yet for attacking the hard and strong, nothing can beat it, There is no one in the whole world who doesn't know it,

And yet there is no one who can put it into practice.

Note: Soft can conquer hard. That is the martial art application of Tai Chi.

So, Tai Chi has put this knowledge into practice!

Page 63

We fire clay and make vessels;

It is precisely where there's no substance, that we find the usefulness of clay pots.

We chisel out doors and windows;

It is precisely in these empty spaces, that we find the usefulness of the room.

Therefore, we regard having something as beneficial;

But having nothing as useful.

Note: Emptiness or nothingness (yielding) is the unique tactic of Tai Chi martial art applications.

Page 66

We look at it but do not see it;

We listen to it but do not hear it;

We touch it but do not hold it;

These three cannot be examined to the limit.

Thus they merge together as one.

"One"- there is nothing more encompassing above it,

And nothing smaller below it.

Boundless, formless! It cannot be named,

And returns to the state of no-thing.

This is called formless form.

This called the beginning of the thread of the Way.

Page 72

Formless am I! Like the ocean;
Shapeless am I! As though I have nothing in which I can rest.
The masses all have their reason for acting;
I alone am stupid and obstinate like a rustic.
But my desires alone differ from those of others—
For I value drawing sustenance from the Mother.

Page 73

As for the nature of the way-it's shapeless and formless.
Formless! Shapeless! Inside there are images.
Shapeless! Formless! Inside there are things.

Note: Formless and shapeless are the ways of Tai Chi. This is what we work so hard to accomplish. We gradually absorb the essence of the forms and shapes we practice into our subconscious. Eventually, every move we make will instinctively follow the way. We are no longer concerned about the Form. We are Formless.

Page 9

When the highest type of men hear the Way, with diligence they're able to practice it;
When average men hear the Way, some things they retain and others they lose; When the lowest type of men hear the Way, they laugh out loud at it.

Note: My teacher Young Wabu often quoted this, describing the three kinds of people he encounters when he presents Classical Tai Chi to them.

Sun-Tzu, *The Art of Warfare*

This book is written by Sun Wu in around 3rd century B.C. I shall quote passages from the following book for discussion.

Sun-Tzu The Art of Warfare

Roger T. Ames, Ballantine Books, New York, 1993

Translated from recently discovered manuscript entombed 140 B. C.

Page 111

So to win a hundred victories in a hundred battles is not the highest excellence; the highest excellence is to subdue the enemy's army without fighting at all.

Note: Tai Chi is basically a defensive martial art following the spirit of the above passage.

Page 115

The expert in battle would first make himself invincible and then wait for the enemy to expose his vulnerability.

Being invincible lies with defense; the vulnerability of the enemy comes with the attack.

Note: This is the strategy of Tai Chi martial art applications. A famous saying about Tai Chi is as follows "If the opponent does not move, I do not move. When opponent prepares to move, I already know how to handle him." That is instinctively you have sensed the weakness in his coming movement.

Page 115

The expert at defense conceals himself in the deepest recesses of the earth; the expert on the attack strikes from out of the highest reaches of the heavens.

Note: In other words, one does not let his defense be visible. Avoid expansive posture which lay open your intent, your strength, and your weakness. When attacking, the force comes from nowhere. That is fajin. The element of surprise is repeatedly emphasized here.

Page 119

Generally in battle use the "straightforward" to engage the enemy and the "surprise" to win the victory. Thus the expert at delivering the surprise assault is as boundless as the heavens and earth, and inexhaustible as the rivers and seas.

Note: That is what my teacher Young Wabu describing how Wu Chian Chuan handled him when they were sparring, continuously keeping him off balance, boundless and inexhaustible. Certainly in this case, Wu was just showing the technique, not seeking a quick victory.

Page 119

There are no more than five cardinal notes, yet in combination, they produce more sounds than could possibly be heard; there are no more than five cardinal colors, yet in combination, they produce more shades and hues than could possibly be seen;.....

"Surprise" and "straightforward" operations give rise to each other endlessly just as a ring is without a beginning or an end.

Page 126

Thus an army does not have fixed strategic advantages or an invariable position. To be able to take the victory by varying one's position according to the enemy's is called being inscrutable.

Note: (Surprising they knew so much about sound and color at such an early time) If one is well versed in the elements of Tai Chi, one should be able to generate infinite variations for the optimum application. This is inscrutable.

Page 123

So veiled and subtle,
To the point of having no form;
So mysterious and miraculous,
To the point of making no sound.
Therefore he can be arbiter of the enemy's fate.

Page 126

The ultimate skill in taking up a strategic position is to have no form. If your position is formless, the most carefully concealed spies will not be able to get a look at it, and the wisest counselors will not be able to lay plans against it.

Note: Avoid expensive, large stance and posture when facing the opponent. It not only exposes your intention but also retards your ability to respond to changing situation. For example, when you have Tight-Compact or small stance, opponent cannot determine where your center of gravity lies. You can shift your weight quickly to engage.

Page 126

…..make him show himself to discover the viability of his battle position; skirmish with him to find out where he is strong and where he is vulnerable.

Page 119

So it is with the expert at battle that his strategic advantage is channeled and his timing is precise. His strategic advantage is like a drawn crossbow and his timing is like releasing the trigger.

Note: Skirmishing and probing the front line and when weak points are discovered, after determination that it is not a trap, marshaling a concentrated force and quickly breaking through the opponent's line and routing the enemy. This kind of scenario plays out all the time in battles. So it is in Tai Chi martial arts application. "Stick to the opponent" is equivalent to skirmishing and probing. Sensing and "ting jin (listen to opponent's power surge and ebb)" is to determine the value of intelligence. Then lightening strike with "fajin".

Page 129

...baiting him with easy gains. Set out after he does, yet arrive before him.

Note: Yielding to opponent to give him easy gain is often used in Tai Chi. If his attack is fully committed with all his momentum. You could give him an "empty" or "nothingness" reception to take full advantage of his momentum. But, if he is cautiously attacking, you have to weigh your neutralization force to give him some satisfaction that he is engaging you with an upper hand, not walking into a trap. This is one of the objectives in push hand training.

Chuang Tzu

Chuang Tzu (Chuangtse) died about 275 B.C. His book has many translated versions, some only translated certain parts of the book. I am using two different translations here.

A Source Book in Chinese Philosophy
The Mystical Way of Chuang Tzu
W. T. Chan, Princeton, 1963

Page 201

...... *Yen Hui saw Confucius again and said "I have made some Progress." "What do you mean?" asked Confucius. "I have Forgotten ceremonies and music" replied Yen Hui. "Very good, but that is not enough" said Confucius. Another day Yen Hui saw Confucius again and said " I have made some progress" "What do you mean?" asked Confucius. Yen Hui said, " I forget everything while sitting down" Confucius' face turned pale. He said, " What do you mean by sitting down and forget everything?"* **"I cast aside my limbs" replied Yen Hui, "discard my intelligence, detached from both body and mind, and become one with Great Universal (Tao). This is called sitting down and forgetting everything."** *Confucius said, "When you become one with the Great Universal you will have no partiality, and when you are part of the process of transformation, you will have no constancy (rigidity). You are really a worthy man. I beg to follow your steps."*

Note: An advanced practitioner essentially discards his intelligence, plays the form subconsciously and conducts his martial arts applications instinctively. He becomes one with the Tao.

The Tao of Tai Chi

The Way of Chuang Tzu

Thomas Merton, New Directions, New York, 1969.

Page 46

A good cook needs a new chopper once a year-he cuts.
A poor cook needs a new one every month-he hacks!

There are spaces in the joints. The blade is thin and keen. When this thinness finds that space, there is all the room you need. It goes like a breeze!

Note: This is how Tai Chi conducts its martial art application. Find the opening (space) in opponent's move, the attack will go like a breeze . In one of the classical writings about Tai Chi has the statement " do not let a fly land on your shoulder"- winning without taking punishment, cutting without dulling the blade.

Page 109

Chi Hsing tze was a trainer of fighting cocks for King Hsuan. He was training a fine bird.

The king kept asking if the bird was ready for combat.

"No not yet," said the trainer. "He is full of fire. He is ready to pick a fight with every other bird. He is vain and confident of his own strength."

.........After ten more days:" Not yet. He still gets that angry look and ruffles his feathers."

Again ten days: The trainer said," Now he is nearly ready. When another bird crows, his eye does not even flicker. He stands immobile....He is a mature fighter..."

Note: There is the saying in classical Tai Chi writing " if the opponent does not move, I remain still. When the opponent is ready to move, I already know how to handle him." This can only be achieved through quietness and sensitivity.

Meng Tzu

Meng Tzu (Mencius, 372-289 BC) is considered to be "the second sage" after Confucius.

I am quoting from the following translation for discussion.

Mencius

Translated by David Hinton

Counterpoint, Washington D. C., 1998

Page 47

The will guides qi, and qi fills the body. So for us the will comes first and qi second............When the will is whole, it moves qi, and when qi is whole, it moves the will. When we stumble and hurry, qi is affected.......

Note: When we practice the Form, we are relaxed except for the flow of internal energy and its associated qi in the torso. The arms are also relaxed during the Form movements without issuing any power from the hand. What is projected into the hands is the martial art intent of the movements. This **intent**, or the **will,** guides the chi to the hands. During actual martial art application, the chi instinctively guides the internal energy or power from the torso to the hands for delivery.

AFTERWORD...

I have spent many years enjoying the beauty and benefits of the treasure of Classical Tai Chi. And spent years uncovering and deciphering the logical foundation that has made this art so precise and practical. To those who have never truly experienced the benefits of practicing Classical Tai Chi, I hope you are intrigued by its possibilities and commit yourself to improving so many aspects of your being by practicing the Forms. To those of you who are starting or have practiced for a while, I know you will have a lifetime of benefits and some of you have or will develop the desire and skills to pass the treasure on so that generations in the future will keep this art alive.

APPENDIX

108 Form Names

1. The preparation Form 太極起式 ....

2. Raise Hands 提手上勢 ....

3. Hand Strums the Lute 手揮琵琶 ....

4. Grasp Peacock's Tail 攬雀尾 ....

5. Single Whip 單鞭 ....

6. Oblique Flying Posture 斜飛勢 ....

7. Raise Hands and Step Up 提手上勢 ....

8. White Crane Spreads Wings 白鶴亮翅 ....

9. Brush Knee Push Step Left & Right 4 Times 摟膝拗步左右四度 ....

10. Hand Strums the Lute 手揮琵琶 ....

11. Step Forward, Deflect, Punch 進步撇攔捶 ....

12. As if Sealed Up 如封似閉 ....

13. Carry Tiger to the Mountain 抱虎歸山 ....

14. Cross Hands 十字手 ....

15. Oblique Brush Knee Push Step 斜摟膝拗步 ....

16. Turn Body Brush Knee Push Step 轉身摟膝拗步 ....

17. Grasp Peacock's Tail 攬雀尾 ....

18. Single Whip 單鞭 ....

19. Fist Under Elbow 肘底看捶 ....

20. Repulse Monkey Left and Right 3 Times 倒撐猴左右三度 ....

41854410R00099

Made in the USA
Lexington, KY
29 May 2015